AF767231

Medical Isotopes

Edited by Syed Ali Raza Naqvi
and Muhammad Babar Imran

Published in London, United Kingdom

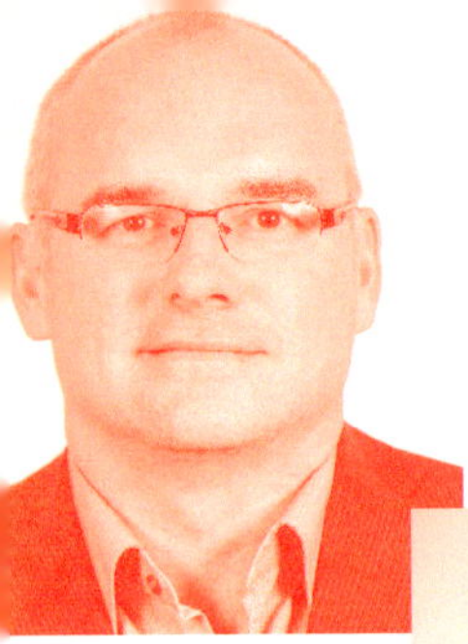
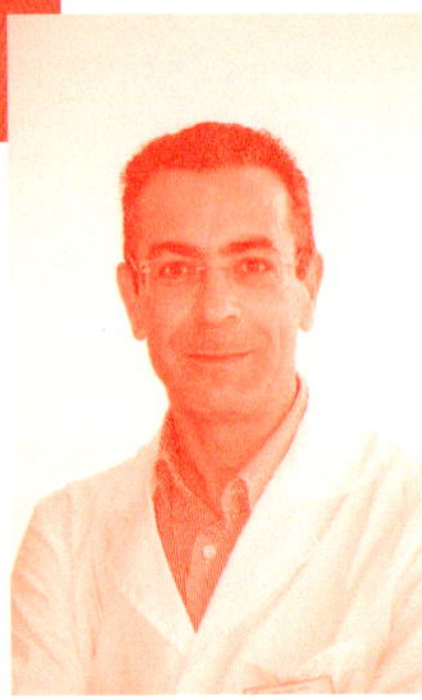
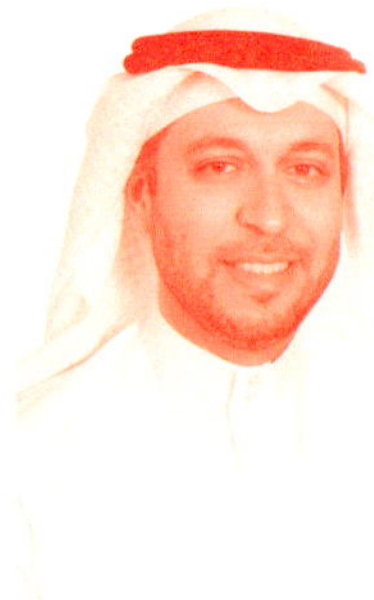
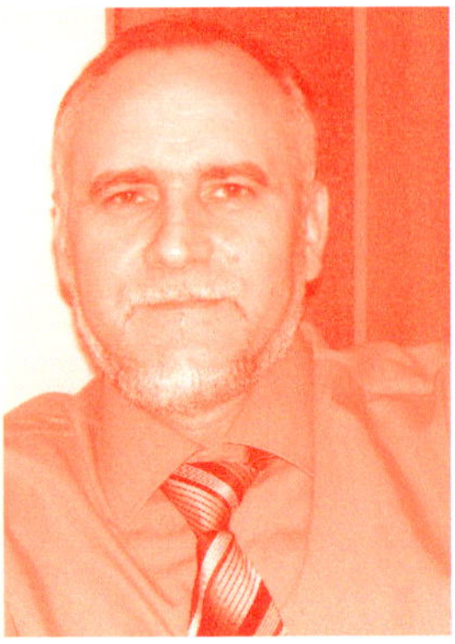
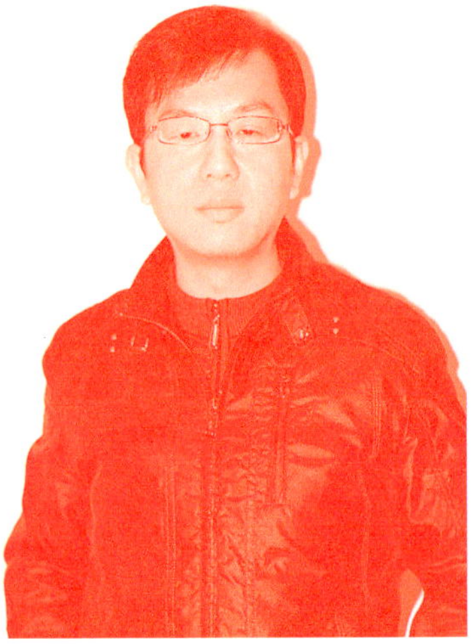
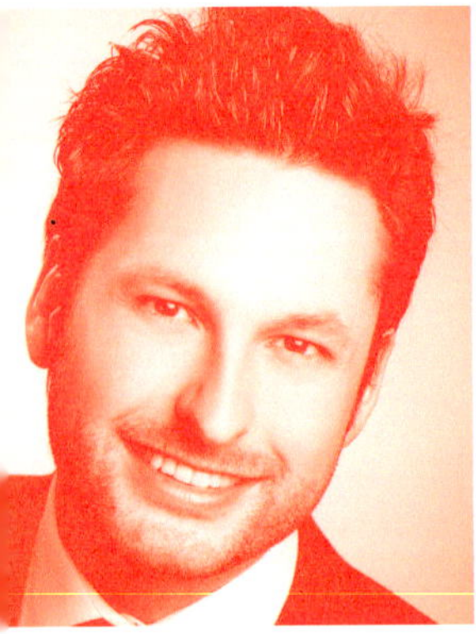
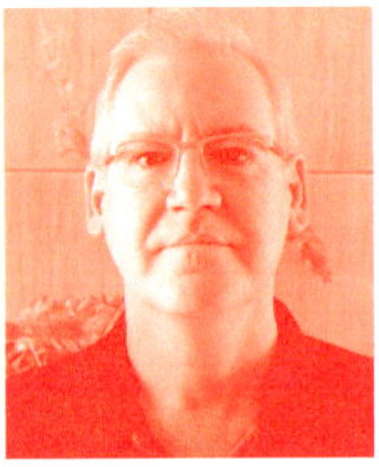

IntechOpen

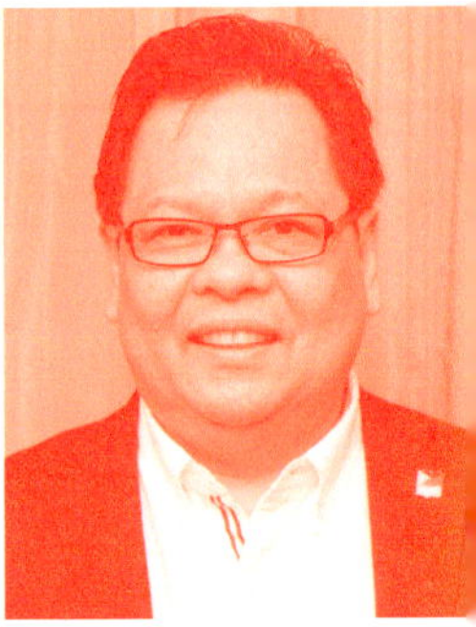
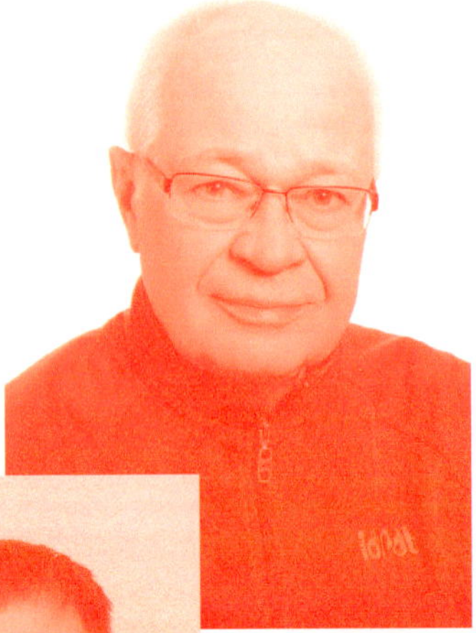
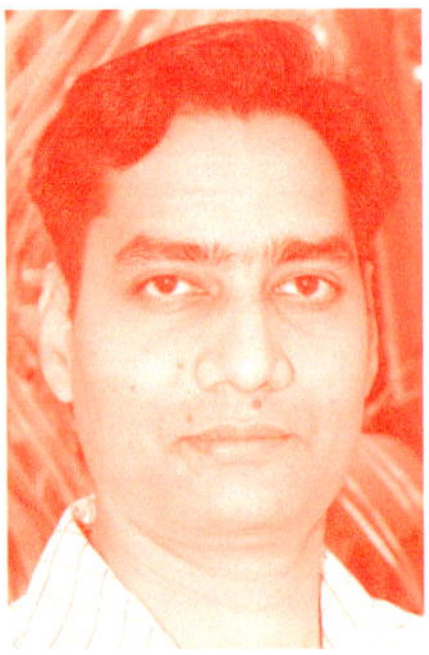
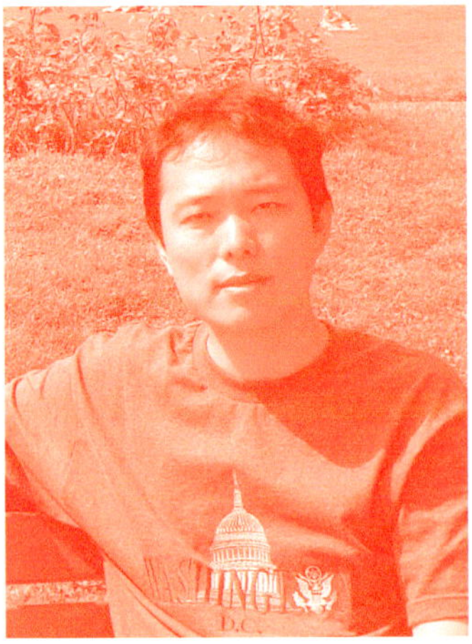
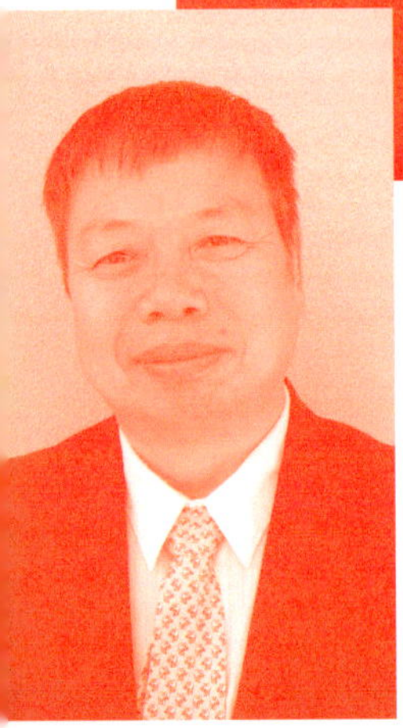
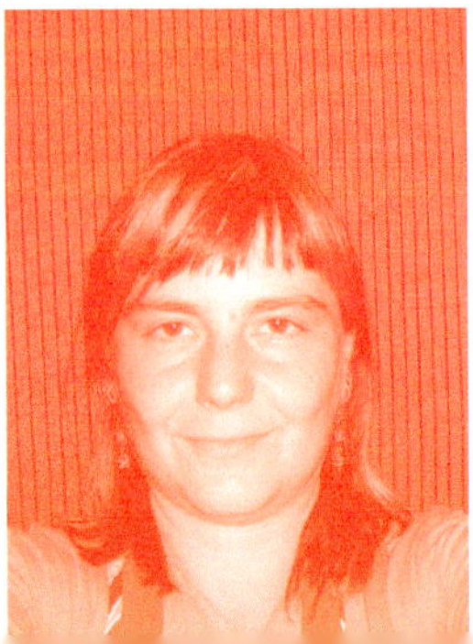

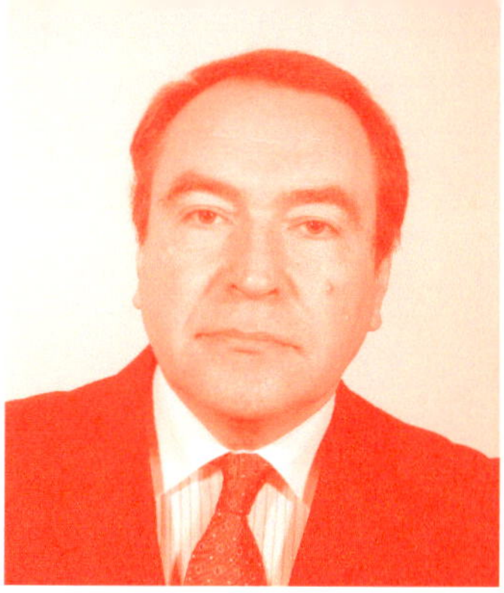
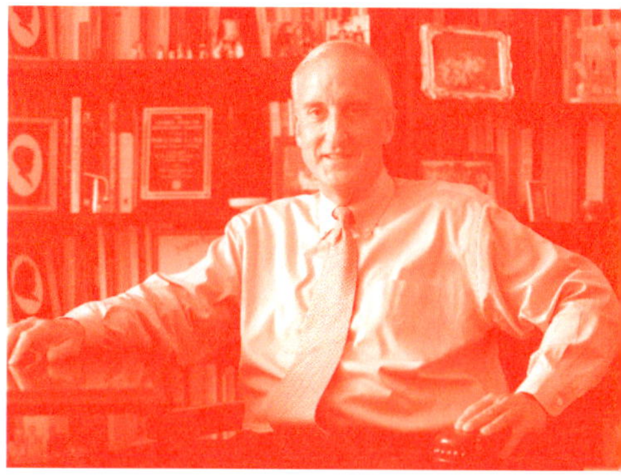
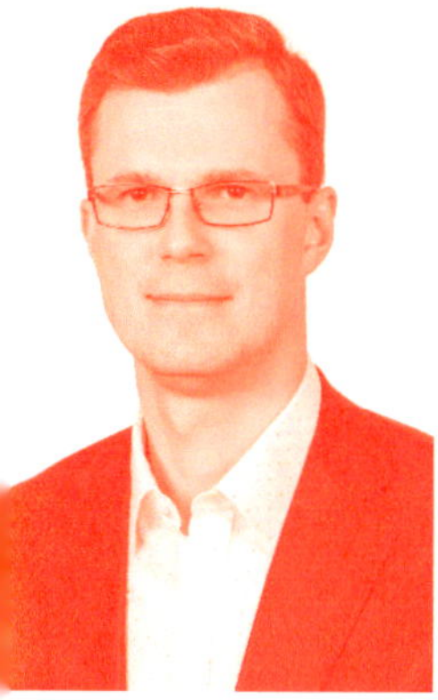
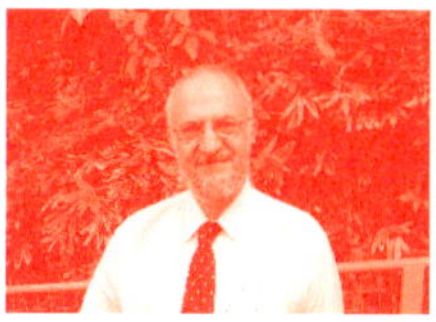
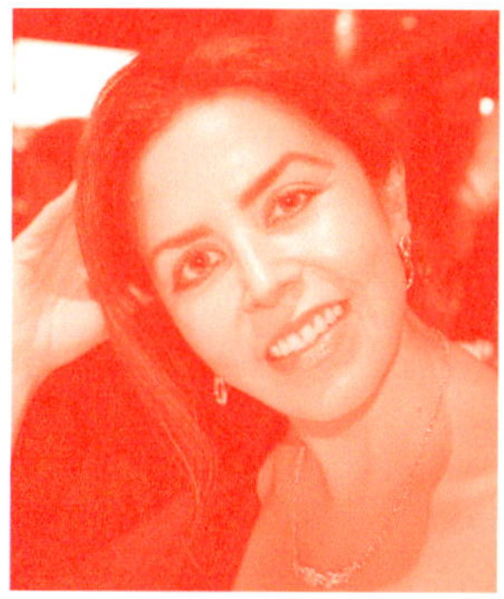

Supporting open minds since 2005

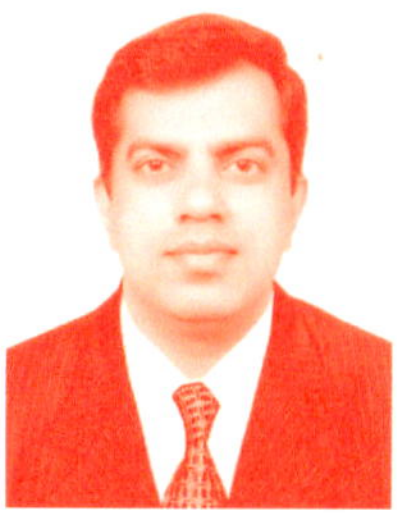
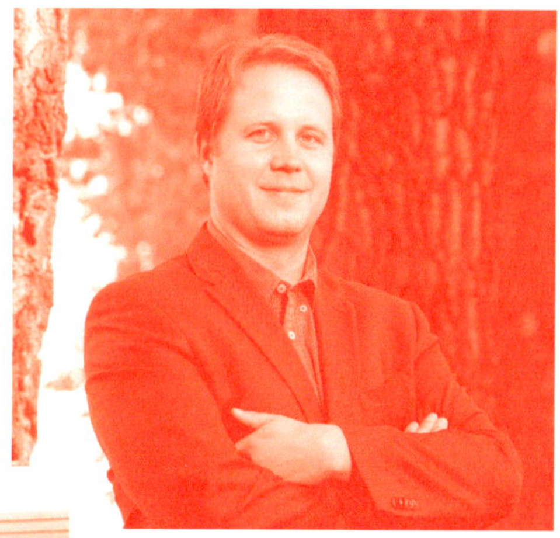
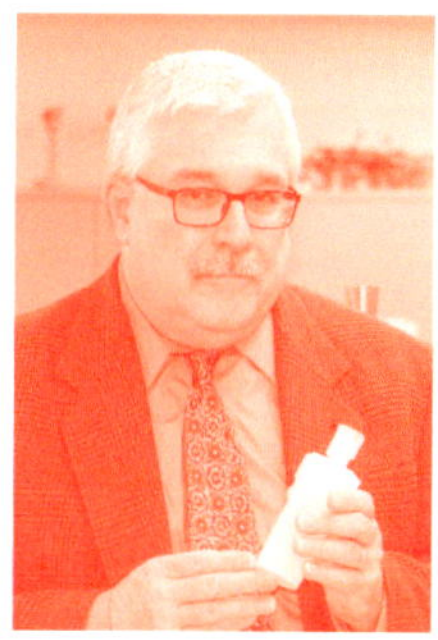
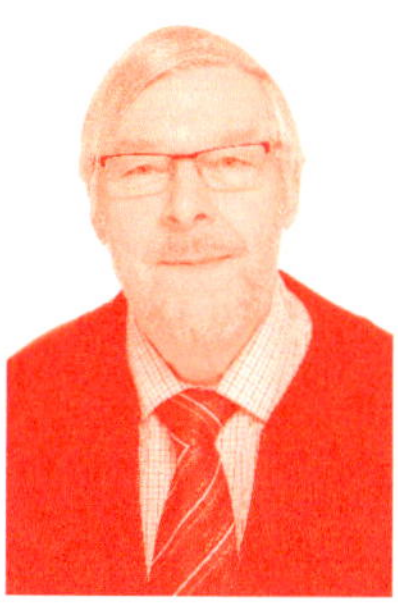
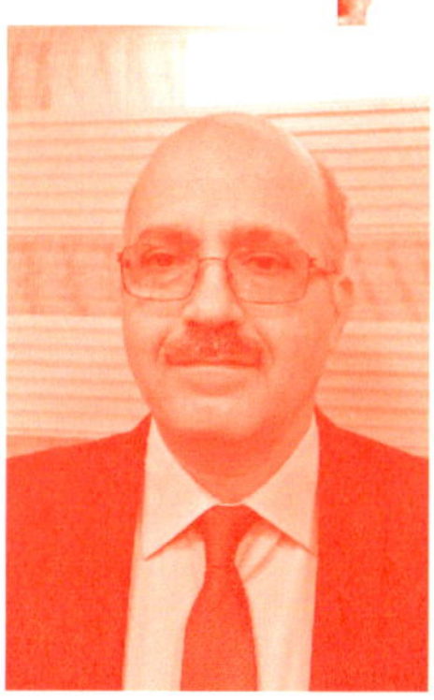
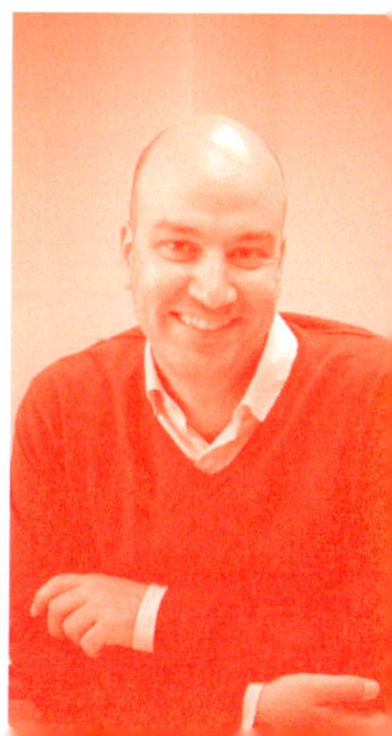
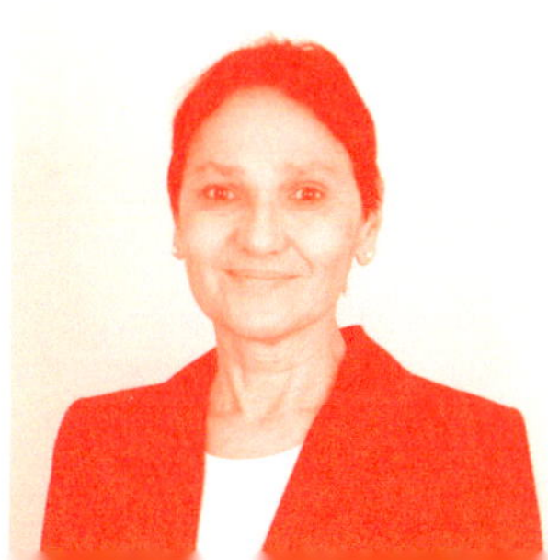

Medical Isotopes
http://dx.doi.org/10.5772/intechopen.77583
Edited by Syed Ali Raza Naqvi and Muhammad Babar Imran

Contributors
Elisabeth Eppard, Yury Saenko, Michael Meisenheimer, Syed Ali Raza Naqvi, Muhammad Babar Imran, Koushlesh Kumar Mishra, Chanchal Deep Kaur, Anil Kumar Sahu, Sarawati Prasad Mishra, Sana Komal, Komal Sarwar, Hijab Umer, Arouma Raza, Zahra Faheem, Samina Roohi, Sana Nadeem, Albena Botushanova, Nikolay Botushanov, Dimple Chopra, Rajnikant Panik, Pankaj Kashyap, Anand Kumar

© The Editor(s) and the Author(s) 2021
The rights of the editor(s) and the author(s) have been asserted in accordance with the Copyright, Designs and Patents Act 1988. All rights to the book as a whole are reserved by INTECHOPEN LIMITED. The book as a whole (compilation) cannot be reproduced, distributed or used for commercial or non-commercial purposes without INTECHOPEN LIMITED's written permission. Enquiries concerning the use of the book should be directed to INTECHOPEN LIMITED rights and permissions department (permissions@intechopen.com).
Violations are liable to prosecution under the governing Copyright Law.

Individual chapters of this publication are distributed under the terms of the Creative Commons Attribution 3.0 Unported License which permits commercial use, distribution and reproduction of the individual chapters, provided the original author(s) and source publication are appropriately acknowledged. If so indicated, certain images may not be included under the Creative Commons license. In such cases users will need to obtain permission from the license holder to reproduce the material. More details and guidelines concerning content reuse and adaptation can be found at http://www.intechopen.com/copyright-policy.html.

Notice
Statements and opinions expressed in the chapters are these of the individual contributors and not necessarily those of the editors or publisher. No responsibility is accepted for the accuracy of information contained in the published chapters. The publisher assumes no responsibility for any damage or injury to persons or property arising out of the use of any materials, instructions, methods or ideas contained in the book.

First published in London, United Kingdom, 2021 by IntechOpen
IntechOpen is the global imprint of INTECHOPEN LIMITED, registered in England and Wales, registration number: 11086078, 5 Princes Gate Court, London, SW7 2QJ, United Kingdom
Printed in Croatia

British Library Cataloguing-in-Publication Data
A catalogue record for this book is available from the British Library

Additional hard and PDF copies can be obtained from orders@intechopen.com

Medical Isotopes
Edited by Syed Ali Raza Naqvi and Muhammad Babar Imran
p. cm.
Print ISBN 978-1-83880-627-9
Online ISBN 978-1-83880-628-6
eBook (PDF) ISBN 978-1-83880-629-3

For EU product safety concerns:
IN TECH d.o.o., Prolaz Marije Krucifikse Kozulić 3, 51000 Rijeka, Croatia, info@intechopen.com or visit our website at intechopen.com.

We are IntechOpen, the world's leading publisher of Open Access books
Built by scientists, for scientists

5,100+
Open access books available

127,000+
International authors and editors

145M+
Downloads

156
Countries delivered to

Our authors are among the
Top 1%
most cited scientists

12.2%
Contributors from top 500 universities

CLARIVATE ANALYTICS BOOK CITATION INDEX INDEXED

WEB OF SCIENCE™

Selection of our books indexed in the Book Citation Index in Web of Science™ Core Collection (BKCI)

Interested in publishing with us?
Contact book.department@intechopen.com

Numbers displayed above are based on latest data collected.
For more information visit www.intechopen.com

Meet the editors

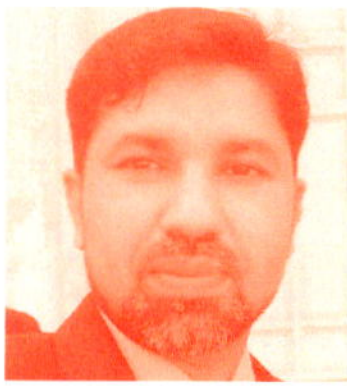

Dr. Naqvi is a radioanalytical chemist and is working as an associate professor of analytical chemistry in the Department of Chemistry, Government College University, Faisalabad, Pakistan. Advance separation techniques, nuclear analytical techniques and radiopharmaceutical analysis are the main courses that he is teaching to graduate and post-graduate students. In the research area, he is focusing on the development of organic- and biomolecule-based radiopharmaceuticals for diagnosis and therapy of infectious and cancerous diseases. Under the supervision of Dr. Naqvi, three students have completed their Ph.D. degrees and 41 students have completed their MS degrees. He has completed three research projects and is currently working on 2 projects entitled "Radiolabeling of fluoroquinolone derivatives for the diagnosis of deep-seated bacterial infections" and "Radiolabeled minigastrin peptides for diagnosis and therapy of NETs". He has published about 100 research articles in international reputed journals and 7 book chapters. Pakistan Institute of Nuclear Science & Technology (PINSTECH) Islamabad, Punjab Institute of Nuclear Medicine (PINM), Faisalabad and Institute of Nuclear Medicine and Radiology (INOR) Abbottabad are the main collaborating institutes.

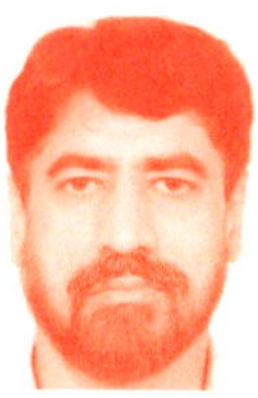

M Babar Imran is a nuclear medicine physician with a special interest in radionuclide theranostics. He is a visiting professor and a faculty member of PIEAS University and the College of Physicians and Surgeons, Pakistan. Dr. Imran has published around 100 research articles, reports, and book chapters. He is the chief editor of the European Journal of Medical Case Reports (http://www.ejmcr.com/) and the Pakistan Journal of Nuclear Medicine (http://pjnmed.com/section/eboard). Dr. Imran has an honor of national and internal awards. He is the only serving nuclear physician at present in this country who has been awarded "Tamgha e Imtiaz" by the President of Pakistan (2006) for his research and academic contribution in the field of nuclear medicine.

Contents

Preface

Currently there are multiple factors in medical history that are playing a pivotal role in reducing the mortality rate in human beings, including diagnosis of hard-to-diagnose diseases from the molecular level to the advanced phase using radioisotopes. Radioisotopes, individually or in tagging with molecule/s to develop radiopharmaceuticals, are practiced clinically either for diagnostic or therapeutic procedures in the field of nuclear medicines. Nuclear medicine has been developed over the past 50 years through a unique partnership among the world laboratories, academia, and industry. The Center for Medicare and Medicaid Services (CMS) reported that nuclear medicine plays an essential role in medical specialties from cardiology to oncology to neurology and it covers a $1.7 billion industry. Further, the Society of Nuclear Medicine estimated that alone in the USA more than 20 million nuclear medicine procedures are performed annually. This book is a brief look into medically interesting radioisotopes and their utilization in the field of nuclear medicine. The book consists of two main sections; "Medical Isotopes Used in SPECT and PET Imaging" and "Nuclear Medicine Mechanism, Imaging and Therapy". The first section comprises of three chapters entitled "Single Photon Emission Computed Tomography (SPECT) Radiopharmaceuticals", "Gallium-68: Radiolabeling of Radiopharmaceuticals for PET Imaging – A Lot to Consider", and "Parathyroid Scintigraphy". While the second section also comprises three chapters entitled "Theranostics – New era in Nuclear Medicine and Radiopharmaceuticals", "Localization Mechanisms of Radiopharmaceuticals", and "Radiolabelled Nanoparticles for Brain Targeting".

Dr. Syed Ali Raza Naqvi
Associate Professor of Radioanalytical Chemistry,
Department of Chemistry,
Government College University,
Faisalabad, Pakistan

Dr. Muhammad Babar Imran (MBBS)
Director of Punjab Institute of Nuclear Medicine,
Faisalabad, Pakistan

Section 1

Medical Isotopes Used in SPECT and PET Imaging

Chapter 1

Single-Photon Emission Computed Tomography (SPECT) Radiopharmaceuticals

Syed Ali Raza Naqvi and Muhammad Babar Imran

Abstract

Nuclear medicine techniques have a great deal of advantage of using gamma radiation emitter radiolabeled compounds to diagnose the long list of infectious and malignant disorders in human systems. The gamma emitter radionuclide-labeled compounds are associated with single photon emission computed tomography (SPECT) camera. SPECT camera mainly offers the detection and analysis of gamma rays origin to furnish the imaging of defective organs in the body. There are about 85% radiopharmaceuticals in clinical practice which are being detected by SPECT camera. The following chapter is an update about the SPECT radiopharmaceuticals that were developed and tried for infection and cancer diagnosis.

Keywords: ^{99m}Tc-antibiotics, SPECT imaging, radiopharmaceuticals, nuclear medicines, infection imaging

1. Introduction

Nuclear medicine technique (NMT) is a detection process that helps in obtaining diagnostic results at molecular level of a disease. The technique is carried out by administrating target-specific radioisotope-labeled organic/biomolecule to patient and collecting the gamma signals through scintillating camera to diagnose the infected organ/tissues. In contrast to advanced instrumental procedures such as magnetic resonance imaging (MRI) and computed tomography (CT) scan, NMT offers a wide range of detection limit. For example, NMT starts working from molecular level when no morphological changes appear; however MRI and CT do this job at the appearance of morphological changes in diseased tissues.

NMT works by administration of radiolabeled molecules (commonly known as radiopharmaceuticals) to patients and acquisition of radiation collected through scintillation camera. There are two main components of radiopharmaceuticals: the organic/biomolecule and the radioisotope. The former approaches diseased cells/tissues and accumulate there at diseased cells and the latter part emits radiation to indicate the position of diseased area.

Diagnosis through NMT means the image of internal body organs like heart, kidney, lungs, breast, brain, bones, tissues, or whole body using γ-emitting radio-pharmaceuticals; for example, indium-111 (^{111}In) and technetium-99m (^{99m}Tc) labeled molecules. These radionuclides are labeled with a variety of compounds including drugs, organic species, peptides, proteins, and antibodies and then

Targeted agent with labeled radiotracer	Emitting radiation	Cancer type/disease
Bombesine indium-111	γ-emitting	Endocrine organ tumor
Pentadecapeptide Technetium-99m	γ-emitting	Breast and prostate cancer, gastro-entero-pancreatic tumors and lung cancer
Oxdronate-^{99m}Tc	γ-emitting	Bones disease
Tilmanocept technetium-99m	γ-emitting	Breast cancer, melanoma and oral Cavity cancer
Pertechnetate technetium-99m	γ-emitting	Urinary and bladder thyroid cancer
Iodinated bombesin I-125	γ-emitting	Endocrine cancer cell growth in endocrine organ breast, prostate, ovaries and testes
Bombesine rhenium-188	γ-emitting	Prostate tumor
FDG-F-18	γ-emitting	Soft tissue cancer and prostate cancer
Oxdronate-^{99m}Tc	γ-emitting	Bones disease

Table 1.
Gamma-emitting radiotracer for diagnostic imaging of different types of cancer and infection [1].

injected into the patient's body. Intravenously administrated radiopharmaceuticals accumulate in specific body part or organ for which it is prepared and scans are obtained by single photon emission computed tomography (SPECT) camera [1]. Scan generated by SPECT camera gives very fruitful information regarding disease and tumor, which makes it easier for doctors to make decision about treatment strategies.

A large number of compounds have been labeled with γ-emitting radiotracers for imaging of different types of cancer and infection. Some of them are shown in **Table 1** below [2].

2. Radiopharmaceuticals

In radiopharmaceuticals, there is a radioactive component which is used for the diagnosis and treatment of different malignancies. Only 5% of radiopharmaceuticals are used for therapeutic purposes while the remaining has diagnostic applications. Radiopharmaceutical has two components: first one is pharmaceutical part and the second is radiotracer as shown in **Figure 1**.

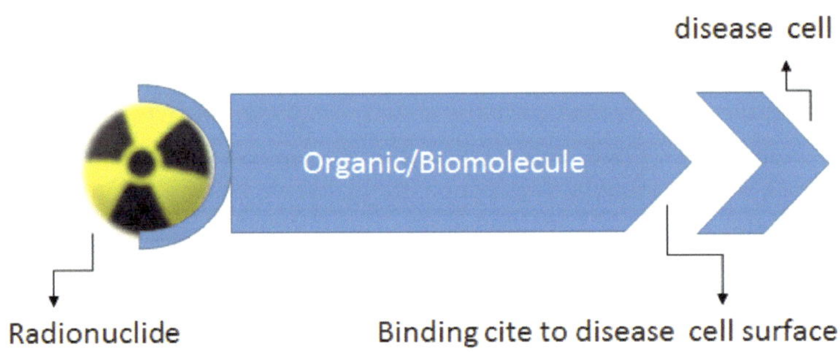

Figure 1.
Radiopharmaceutical and its design.

Targeted agent with labeled radiotracer	Emitting radiation	Cancer type/disease
Metastron ($^{89}SrCl_2$)	β-emitting	Skeletal cancer
Radium-223 dichloride	α-emitting	Bone metastasis, breast and prostate cancer
Samarium-153-EDTMP	β-emitting	Bone and prostate cancer

Table 2.
Commonly used radiopharmaceuticals for therapeutic purpose [4].

Effectiveness of the radiopharmaceutical depends upon both parts. In order to prepare a good and efficient radiopharmaceutical, the first step involves the selection of a pharmaceutical component which is very critical [3]. Pharmaceuticals that have a preferable accumulation in targeted body organ, tissues, or cells should be selected. After the selection of pharmaceutical component, pharmaceutical is labeled with a suitable radiotracer. The radiopharmaceutical is subjected to administration after a routine quality control procedure. There are many disease targeted radiolabeled agents or compounds that are commonly used for diagnosis and therapeutic purpose. From diagnostic point of view, disease-targeted agents (either a drug or any other compound) are labeled with γ-emitting radiotracer, and for therapeutic purpose, these agents are labeled with β and α radiotracer like lutetium-177 (^{177}Lu) and Yatrium-90 (^{90}Y) [4]. In **Table 2**, some of the disease-targeted agents (radiopharmaceuticals) are shown which are used for diagnostic imaging and therapeutic purpose of different diseases and cancers.

3. SPECT—radiopharmaceuticals

Radiopharmaceuticals which are used to diagnose the cancer and infection by using the γ-emitting radionuclides such as ^{111}In and ^{99m}Tc are known as SPECT radiopharmaceuticals. The radiotracer which is used for diagnostic purposes should have following properties [5]:

- Easy availability at nuclear medicine center
- Low cost
- Short effective half-life then labeled pharmaceutical
- Carrier free
- Nontoxic

γ-emitting radiotracer	Half-life (hours)	Generator	Gamma energy	Abundance of γ-emission (%age)
Indium-111	67.32	Cyclotron	0.171 MeV 0.245 MeV	90.5 94
Technetium-99m	6.02	$^{99m}Mo/^{99m}Tc$	140 keV	88.9
Iodine-123	13.22	Cyclotron	159 keV	82.8

Table 3.
Common properties of γ-emitting radionuclides.

- Free from α and β particles emission (with little emission)
- Biological half-life not greater than time of study
- Suitable energy range
- Chemically reactive to form coordinate covalent bonds with the compound which is to be labeled

Common properties of γ-emitting radionuclides for SPECT imaging are given in **Table 3**.

4. Characteristic of technetium-99m for labeling

More than 85% of radiopharmaceuticals which are being used to diagnose the cancer and infection are ^{99m}Tc labeled. The reason for using the ^{99m}Tc is due to following characteristics:

- Half-life of technetium is 6 hours which is sufficient to examine the catabolic as well as anabolic processes which occur in patient and minimal radiation exposure time to the patients [6].
- Energy of the γ-rays emitted by technetium is very low (140 keV) which does not greatly damage the soft tissues of the patient body, although they have low energy but can be detected by any sensitive gamma camera [7].
- Its excretion rate from the patient body is very fast.
- Its short half-life enables us to get the imaging information very quickly.
- Technetium is very reactive to make complex with compounds.
- Decay of technetium takes place through isomeric transitions due to which electrons and gamma radiation of low energy is emitted. Therefore, beta radiation exposure to patent is negligible.
- Due to the emission of same energy levels of gamma radiation, the detector alignment becomes very accurate as no beta radiation is emitted.
- Most important property of technetium is that its oxidation state can be changed according to the desired targeted body organ and parts, which makes it possible to develop a biological technetium labeled compound which can accumulate in high amount on that targeted organ and part of body which is under investigation [8].

5. Chemistry of ^{99m}Tc and oxidation state for labeling

Technetium belongs to transition metal family; its electronic configuration and physical properties are shown in table given below (**Table 4**). There are 22 isotopes of the technetium, but none of them is stable in nature. Half-life of ^{99}Tc is 0.25 million years in its ground state. Oxidation state of technetium varies from −3 to +7 as shown in **Table 4** below. This happens due to the 4d and 5s loss or gain of

Properties of technetium	Values
Atomic number	43
Atomic mass (amu)	98
Electronic configuration	$1s^2,2s^2,2p^6,3s^2,3p^6,3d^{10},4s^2,4p^6,4d^6,5s^1$
Density gm/cm^3 (at 25°C)	11.5
Oxidation state	−3, −1, 0, +1,+2,+3,+4,+5,+6,+7 (+4 and +7 are more stable)
Melting point in Kelvin	2430.15
Boiling point in Kelvin	5150.15
Occurrence	Solid state (naturally)
Electronagetivity	1.9
First, second, and third ionization energy (kJ/mol)	702, 1472, and 2850, respectively
Electron affinity (kJ/mol)	58
Heat of vaporization kJ/mol	660
Group	VIIB (7)
Metal category	Transitions metal
Period	Fifth
Color	Silvery gray
Numbers of isotopes	Twenty-two

Table 4.
Physical and chemical properties of technetium.

electrons by 4d orbital. Different types of ligands which are used to label the technetium and chemical conditions under which labeling process is accomplished are responsible for steadiness of such types of oxidation state. It is observed that technetium is found in nature in the form of halides (TcF_6, $TcCl_6$ and $TcBr_4$, oxide, [TcO_2, Tc_2O_7], sulfides [Tc_2S_7], and pertechnetate $^{99m}TcO_4^-$ in +4 to +7 oxidation states). Oxidation states of smaller values such as −1, +2, +3 are naturally stabilized during complex formation with varieties of ligands; for example, +3 oxidation state is stabilized by the chelating agent, methylene diphosphate [9]. Without the use of these chelating agents in complex formation, the oxidation state will not remain constant and technetium would oxidize to +4 oxidation state and eventually change to +7 oxidation state which is most stable state in complex. The +5 and +6 oxidation of technetium is habitually charged to +4 and +7 oxidation states as shown in the following Eqs. 1 and 2 which is most stable regardless of their proportion.

$$3Tc^{+5}\ 2Tc^{+4+}\ Tc^{+7} \tag{1}$$

$$3Tc^{+6}\ Tc^{+4} + 2Tc^{+7} \tag{2}$$

The coordination number of the technetium during complex formation can be changed between 4 and 9.

6. Reducing agents and reduction of $^{99m}TcO_4^-$

Technetium generated by Moly generator presents in the form of sodium-pertechnetate (^{99m}Tc-$NaTcO_4$). In this pertechnetate ion, the oxidation state of technetium is +7 and structure of the $^{99m}TcO_4^-$ is pyramid tetrahedron in which Tc atom is present in the center of the tetrahedron with +7 oxidation state and four oxygen atoms located at the apexes of the triangular pyramid. This geometry and oxidation state is identical to the permanganate ion MnO_4^- and perrhenate ion ReO_4^- ion. Structure of the pertechnetate ion TcO_4^- is shown in **Figure 2**.

Pertechnetate $^{99m}TcO_4$ is a nonreactive molecule and cannot be used directly for labeling; therefore, it is necessary to reduce the pertechnetate from +7 oxidation state to lower oxidation state for labeling purposes. For the reduction of the pertechnetate $^{99m}TcO_4$ form +7 oxidation state to lower oxidation state, a variety of reducing agents are employed such as stannous citrate ($C_{12}H_{10}O_{14}Sn_3$), stannous tartrate ($C_4H_4O_6Sn$), stannous chloride ($SnCl_2.2H_2O$), concentrated hydrochloric acid (HCl), dithionite ($O_4S_2^{-2}$), ferrous sulfate ($FeSO_4$), and sodium boro tetrahdride ($NaBH_4$). However, the most frequently used reducing agent in labeling of the compounds with technetium process is stannous chloride dihydrate ($SnCl_2.2H_2O$) [10]. Electrolysis can also be utilized as a method for reducing sodium-pertechnetate (^{99m}Tc-$NaTcO_4$) and use zirconium as an anode and labeling compound. However, following common characteristics are being considered to choose a reducing agent in ^{99m}Tc chemistry.

- It should give effectual reduction at compassionate pH environment.
- It should have long shelf life mean remain unaffected when they are stored for long time.
- It should not incorporate within the final product of the complex.
- It should give well-defined oxidation state in order to generate intrinsic complex.
- It should not interfere with complex formation procedure.

Reduction of pertechnetate $^{99m}TcO_4$ with the help of stannous chloride is accomplished in acidic medium, and reaction is given below.

$$3Sn^{+2}\ 3Sn^{+4} + 6\ e \quad (3)$$

$$2^{99m}TcO_4 + 16H^+ + 6e^{99m}Tc^{+4} + 8H_2O \quad (4)$$

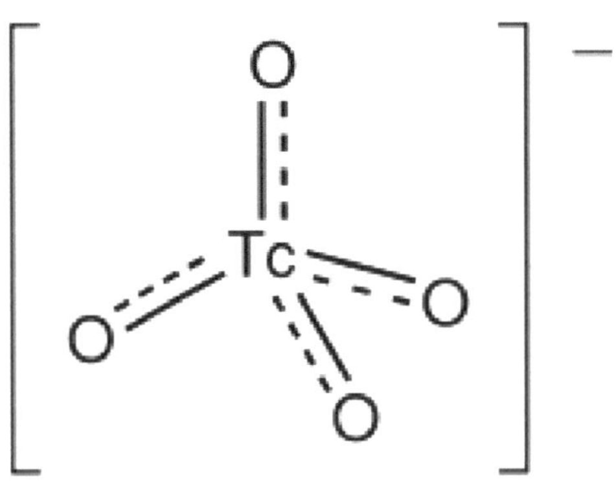

Figure 2.
Structure of pertechnetate ion $^{99m}TcO_4^-$.

Overall reaction

$$2^{99m}TcO_4 + 16H^+ + 3Sn^{+2}\ {}^{99m}Tc^{+4} + 8H_2O + 3Sn^{+4} \quad (5)$$

It is clear from the Eq. 4 that technetium reduces from higher oxidation state +7 to lower oxidation state +4. Under different chemical and physical conditions, other oxidation state of ^{99m}Tc such as $^{99m}Tc^{+3}$ and $^{99m}Tc^{+5}$ are likely to be formed or a mixture of all these oxidation states could possibly exist. Stannous chloride as a reducing agent is usually used in a very small amount while ^{99m}Tc is commonly administrated in the concentration $\sim 10^{-9}$ M.

7. Labeling of chelating agents with reduce technetium

Technetium-99m after reduction forms reactive species and attains the ability to bind with a variety of chelating agents to generate the labeled product. In order to form the additive bond, normally, chelating agent donates the lone pairs of the electrons to make coordinate covalent bond with ^{99m}Tc. Compounds containing the electron donating group such as carboxylic group (—COOH), amines ($—NH_{2)}$, hydroxyl (—OH), and thiol group (—SH) are good chelates such as DTPA (diethylenetriamine pentaacetic acid) and gluceptate.

8. Oxidation state of technetium for labeling

Technetium is found in variable oxidation states ranging from −1 to +7, but it frequently forms complexes in +5 oxidation state. A number of technetium complexes with other oxidation states also exist in increasing order [10]. Complex of technetium in +6, +2 and zero oxidation state are not synthesized because they are not fruitful for medical purpose. Different complexes of technetium that they from in different oxidation states are as follows:

- Complex of technetium in +7 oxidation state (Tc^{+7}). Technetium naturally occurs in this state, and it is most stable and nonreactive toward any chelating agent in this oxidation state. Technetium in +7 oxidation state is found in the form of technetium heptasulfide and pertechnetate $^{99m}TcO_{4.}$

- Complex of technetium in +5 oxidation state (Tc^{+5}). Technetium is present in this oxidation state in the form of complexes such as^{99m}Tc-gluconate, ^{99m}Tc-glucepetate, and ^{99m}Tc-citrate. During these complexes formation, reduction of technetium (pertechnetate $^{99m}TcO^-{}_4$) from +7 oxidation state to lower oxidation state +5 is accomplished with stannous chloride in an aqueous medium. It is observed that technetium in +5 oxidation state have tendency to form the complex with sulfur containing molecules (dithiols) in solid state. In these sulfur complexes, four sulfur atoms are located at the corner of the square planes and oxygen atom at the apex of square pyramid. Compounds with six coordination number are preferably formed in the aqueous medium, and molecules exhibit more stable structure in the form of octahedral geometry. Diaminodithiol (DATA) is one of the best examples of such compounds. In these complexes, oxidation state of technetium is +5 and complexes are neutral and stable in this oxidation state.

- Complex of technetium in +4 oxidation state (Tc^{+4}). Oxidation state of technetium in complexes of TcO_2 and hexahalo is +4. The reducing agent which is used to reduce the pertechnetate $^{99m}TcO_4$ from +7 oxidation state to lower oxidation state +4 ($TcO2.xH_2O$) is zinc with HCl. However, 20% of technetium reduces to technetium metal by this method. In technetium-99m-hydroxyethylidene diphosphonate (HEDP) complex, it is observed that the oxidation state of technetium is changeable which is highly dependent upon the pH of the method which is used to synthesize the complex. In acidic medium, the oxidation state of technetium is +3; in alkaline medium, it is +5; and in neutral medium, it is +4 [11]. This means that a slight change in pH can change the oxidation state of technetium pointing to the fact that they may exist as a mixture of all oxidation states like +3, +5 and +4 in technetium-99m-hydroxyethylidene diphosphonate (HEDP) complex.

- Complex of technetium in +3 oxidation state (Tc^{+3}). A number of technetium-99m complexes exist with +3 oxidation state in acidic medium. These complexes include DTPA (diethylenetriamine pentaacetic acid, ethylenediamine tetraacetic acid (EDTA), DMSA (dimercaptosuccinic acid) and hepatobiliary iminodiacetic acid. However, the oxidation state of technetium in the complex EDTA and DTPA become +4 in alkaline as well as in neutral medium. A variety of technetium complexes in which technetium exists in +3 oxidation state are used for myocardial scanning. These include complexes of technetium-99m with phosphine, arsine and BATOs (boronic acid adduct of technetium dioxime comples).

- Complex of technetium in +1 oxidation state (Tc^{+1}). This oxidation state is stabilized with the help of coordinate covalent bond with different types of ligands in aqueous medium. In this oxidation state, compounds are usually stable in water and air.

9. Chemistry of indium and oxidation state for labeling

Indium belongs to aluminum which are naturally occurring transition metals. Its chemical and physical properties are enlisted in **Table 5**. Indium is a soft silvery white metal which is not found in free elemental form but found in the form of combined state such as halides $InCl_3$, $InBr_3$ InI_3 and InF_3, sulphide and oxide (In_2O_3). Indium exists in three oxidation state +3, +2 and +1 but indium in +3 oxidation state it appears more stable. Thirty-nine isotopes of indium have been reported but only three isotopes such as indium-111, indium-113 and indium-115 are commonly found. Indium-111 with half-life of 66.32 hours are used in radiopharmaceutical for imaging purpose

Properties of indium	Values
Atomic number	49
Atomic mass (amu)	114.818
Electronic configuration	$1s^2,2s^2,2p^6,3s^2,3p^6,3d^{10},4s^2,4p^6,4d^{10},5s^2,5p^1$
Density gm/cm^3 (at 25°C)	7.31
Oxidation state	+1,+2,+3, (+3 more stable)
Melting point in Kelvin	429.75
Boiling point in Kelvin	2353.15
Occurrence	Solid state (naturally)
Electronegativity	1.78

Properties of indium	Values
First, second and third ionization energy (kJ/mol)	558, 1820, 2704, respectively
Electron affinity (kJ/mol)	29
Heat of vaporization kJ/mol	23.2
Group	IIIA (13)
Metal category	Poor metal (posttransitional)
Period	5th
Color	Silvery white
Natural isotopes (two)	Indium-113 and Indium-115
Artificial isotope	39 in number but Indium-111 and Indium-113 are important

Table 5.
Physical and chemical properties of indium.

[12]. γ-radiation emitted by indium-111 have an energy of 247 keV and 172 keV and the percentage of γ-radiation emitted by indium-111 is 90.6% with minimal β-radiation emission that make the indium −111 a good imaging radiotracer.

These γ-emitting radionuclide labeled compounds can be utilized to identify the exact position and location of the infection in different parts and organs such as brain, arteries, joints, bones and tissues. In **Table 6**, a number of compounds bound

Sr no.	Labeled compound	Labeled radioisotope	SPECT imaging model	Pathology	Sensitivity/ accuracy	Refs.
1.	Oxyquinolone-labeled leukocytes	^{111}In	Human model		90%	[1]
2.	Exametazime-labeled leukocytes	^{99m}Tc	Human model	Reticuloendothelialsystem visualization	90%	[1]
	Sulfur colloid	^{99m}Tc	Human model	osteomyelitis		
3.	Methylene diphosphonate	^{99m}Tc	Human model		High sensitivity low specificity	[2]
4.	Labeled leukocytes	^{111}In	Human model			[2]
5.	HMPAO labeled leukocytes	^{99m}Tc	Human model			[2]
6.	Biotin	^{111}In	Human model	Spinal infection	93%	[2]
7.	UBI	^{99m}Tc	Human model	Soft tissue and bone infection	95%	[3]
8.	MDP	^{99m}Tc	Human model	Marrow imaging		[4]
9.	HMPAO-labeled leukocyte	^{99m}Tc	Human model	Prosthetic joint infections	91%	[5]

Table 6.
General radiopharmaceuticals developed based on SPECT imaging.

with γ-emitting radionuclides (indium-111 and technetium-99m) along with their sensitivity and imaging purpose are shown.

10. Methods of radiolabeling

The radiolabeling of antibiotics, drugs, peptides, proteins and organic species with different radiotracer has increased reasonably from imaging point of view in medical, biochemical and other associated fields. In the field of medical imaging, compounds are labeled with two types of radionuclides: (a) compound labeled with those radionuclide that emitted the gamma radiation and have large number of application and especially used for in vivo imaging of a number of organs and (b) secondly, the compounds are labeled with radionuclide that emitted the β-radiation and have limited in vitro study and therapeutic treatment of the disease site. During the labeling process of a compound with a radiotracer, atoms or group of atoms of compound are replaced by different or similar atoms or group of atoms of the radiotracers [13]. In order to obtain, certain type of the labeling, the labeling process is carried out under constant conditions of temperature, pressure and incubation time. There are mainly six methods for labeling of the compound with radiotracer as shown in **Table** 7.

Isotopic exchange	Labeling of the compounds with C-14, S-35, I-135 labeling of T3 and T4 and H-3.
Labeling with bifunctional Chelating Agent	In-111 DTPA albumin Tc-99m DTPA antibody
Introduction of foreign label	Labellng of the proteins with I-125. Tc-99m labeled radiopharmaceuticals Labeling of the hormones with I-125 Labeling of the cells with In-111 F-18 fluorodeoxyglucose
Biosynthesis	Labeling of the compounds with C-14 Co-57 cyanocobalamin Se-75 selenomethionine
Excitation labeling	Labeling of the compounds with I-223 from Xe-123 decay Labeling of the compounds with Br-77 from Kr-77 decay
Recoil labeling	Iodinated compounds Compounds label with H-3

Table 7.
Methods for labeling of the compound with radiotracers [13].

11. Direct method labeling without bi-functional chelating agent

In this type of labeling process, there is no need of bi-functional chelating agents or metal cheater. These are discussed below.

11.1 Isotopes exchange labeling

In this method, some atoms from the compound which is to be labeled is replaced by isotope of the same atom of the element having different atomic mass (more or less) such as I-123, I-124, I-125, I-127, and I-131. the compound is labeled with isotope of the same element so the compound to be labeled and radiolabeled are similar in biological properties, except for the energy emitted from different isotopes of the same element which is used for labeling [14]. This method used for in vitro study. Examples of isotope exchange labeling reactions are labeling of the triiodothyronine (T3) with I-125, labeling of thyroxine with I-125, and labeling with C-14, S-35 and H-3 labeled compounds [15].

11.2 Introduction of a foreign label

In this process of labeling, a molecule of known biological function is labeled with a radionuclide. This labeling occurs by forming covalent bond or co-ordinate covalent bond. The attaché radiotracer is unknown (foreign) to the molecule, and labeling does not occur due to the exchange of its isotope. In most of these types of compounds, chelation is the cause for bond formation. In such bonds, more than one atom donates a pair of electrons to the foreign acceptor atom that is mostly a transition metal. Majority of Tc-99m labeled compounds are developed by this process such as binding of Tc-99m with DTPA, gluceptate, etc.

11.3 Biosynthesis

The biosynthesis method involves the growth of the microorganisms in a culture medium that contains the radiotracer. When microorganisms (bacteria) grow in such a medium, the radiotracer is introduced into the metabolites that are produced by the metabolic activity of the organism. This metabolite is then chemically separated. Example of such product is preparation of ^{57}Co-B12 by using a bacterium *Streptomyces griseus*.

11.4 Recoil labeling

It is of limiting interest and cannot be preceded on large scale for labeling because it has low specific activity of the bounded molecule. The method involves generation of recoil ions or atoms as particles are emitted by the nucleus. These generated atoms or ions then form a bond with the targeted molecule. This high energy of recoil atoms gives poor yield.

11.5 Excitation labeling

Radioactive and very reactive daughter ions that are produced by nuclear decay process are used in excitation labeling process. In β-decay and electron capture processes, there is a production of highly energetic charged particle ions which have the ability to label the compound of interest. When Kr-77 undergoes the decay process, it yields Br-77. These (Br-77) energetic ions are able to bind the compound of interest when exposed to it [16]. A number of proteins are labeled with I-123 when protein is exposed to Xe-123 which decays into energetic I-123 and label the protein. Main disadvantage of this method is poor yield.

12. Indirect method labeling using bi-functional chelating agent

A chelating agent is a substance that has the ability to form multiple bonds with a single metal ion, thus acts as a multidendate ligand. Bi-functional chelating agent is that which has two are more separate covalent or coordinate covalent bonds with a ligand which is polydendate in nature. The labeling process using bi-functional chelating agent involves the bond formation at two sites: one bond is formed by the bi-functional chelating agent with macromolecule such as protein and antibody and other bond is formed with metal ion such as Tc-99m. There are many bi-functional chelating agents being used currently; however, most important are diethylene-triamine pentaacetic acid (DTPA), metallothionein, diamide dimercaptide (N_2S_2), dithiosemicarbazone, and hydrazinonicotinamide.

There are two types of labeling process by using bi-functional chelating agent.

(a) Tc-99m chelate method: In this method, a chemical is used to carry out chelation (such as diamidodithiol and cyclam) and labeling of macromolecules such as protein by forming the bond between chelating agent and protein (macromolecule).

(b) Indirect chelater antibody method: In this method, bi-functional chelating agent forms a bond with macromolecule and then it reacts with metal ion to form the complex known as metal-chelator-macromolecule complex. By using indirect chelator antibody method, a number of antibodies are labeled. The biological function of the antibodies may be affected due to the presence of the chelating agent; therefore, it is necessary to check the labeling products before a clinical trial. It is no doubt that the prelabeled chelating method gives pure metal-chelate- complex with precise structural study. However, the main drawback of this method is that it is a lengthy procedure and gives poor yield [17].

These SPECT-radiopharmaceuticals can also be developed for early and accurate diagnosis of cancer in different body parts and organs. A variety of drugs and compounds such as peptides, proteins, antibodies, and organic species were labeled with radionuclides such as indium-111 and technetium-99m, and these radiolabeled compounds are used for the successful and accurate diagnosis of different types of cancer in human and mice models [18]. In **Table 8**, a number of compounds which

Sr. no.	Labeled compound	Labeled radioisotope	SPECT imaging model	Pathology	Sensitivity/ accuracy	Refs.
1.	Anti-PSMA nanobody	^{111}In	Human model	Tumor target		[6]
2.	HYNIC-Glu-Urea	^{99m}Tc	Human model	Metastatic prostate cancer		[6]
5.	DTPA-AMB8LK	^{111}In	Mice model	Pancreatic cancer	23.6 ± 3.9% ID/g	[7]
6.	Octreotide	^{111}In	Human model	Neuroendocrine tumor (NETs)	95%	[8]
7.	Sestamibi	^{99m}Tc	Human model	Parathyroid adenoma	Range from 85 to 95%	[8]
8.	MDP	^{99m}Tc	Human model	Bone metastases	Very sensitive	[8]
9.	(Arg11)CCMSH	^{99m}Tc	Mice model	Murine melanoma	3.33 ± 0.50% ID/g	[9]
10.	DOTA-Re(Arg11) CCMSH	^{111}In	Mice model	Murine melanoma	8.19 ± 1.63% ID/g	[9]
11.	DTPA-octreotide	^{111}In	Mice model	Lung cancer	Bm/B was 3.1 ± 0.6	[19]
12.	HYNIC-TOC	^{99m}Tc	Human model	Metastatic neuroendocrine tumors	Sensitivity 87%	[10]
13.	DTPA-octreotide	^{111}In	Mice model	Somatostatin-receptor tumors: evaluation	4.3%ID/g	[11]

Sr. no.	Labeled compound	Labeled radioisotope	SPECT imaging model	Pathology	Sensitivity/ accuracy	Refs.
14.	HYNIC-TOC	^{99m}Tc	Mice model	Somatostatin-receptor tumors: evaluation	5.8 ± 9.6% ID/g	[11]
15.	HMPAO	^{99m}Tc	Mice model	Neuroblastoma	88%	[12]
16.	Oxine	^{111}In	Mice model	Neuroblastoma	80%	[12]
17.	Rhenium sulfide colloidal nanoparticles	^{99m}Tc	Rabbit model	Sentinel lymph node	Radiolabeled 98.5 ± 0.5%	[13]
18.	TDMPP complex	^{111}In	Mice model	Tumor imaging		[14]
19.	DOTA conjugate - TA138	^{111}In	Mouse model	Tumor imaging	9.39% ID/g	[15]

Table 8.
SPECT-radiopharmaceuticals using Tc-99m and In-111 for cancer imaging.

are labeled with γ-emitting radiotracer for SPECT imaging of different types of cancer with accuracy are shown.

SPECT-radiopharmaceuticals are not only used to identify infections and malignancies but are equally used to know the effectiveness of the treatment strategy which is used to cure the infections and tumors. That means, we can employ the SPECT-radiopharmaceuticals for follow-up strategy to know about the effectiveness of a treatment methods. A large numbers of radiolabeled compounds are being used to identify the effects of previous treatment strategy, for example, pentetreotide is labeled with indium-111 to follow-up of the neuroendocrine tumor therapy (tumor generated due to the hormonal cell and nerves system) in gastrointestinal tract, lungs, pancreas, and rest of the body (**Table 9**).

Sr no.	Labeled compound	Labeled radioisotope	SPECT imaging model	Pathology	Sensitivity/ accuracy	Refs.
1	Nano-colloids	^{99m}Tc	Human model	Breast cancer and melanomas	Well accepted	[16]
2	Radio-colloid	^{99m}Tc	Human model	Breast cancer, head/neck malignancies, prostate cancer and gynecological malignancies		[16]
3	Pentetreotide	^{111}In	Human model	Neuroendocrine tumors	95%	[16]
4	Capromab	^{111}In	Human model	Biochemical disease-free survival and disease-specific survival in primary prostate cancer	46%	[16]
5	Medronate	^{99m}Tc	Human model	Bone imaging		[16]
6	Labeled white blood cells	^{111}In	Human model	Inflammation imaging		[16]
7	Labeled white blood Cells	^{99m}Tc	Human model	Inflammation imaging		[16]

Sr no.	Labeled compound	Labeled radioisotope	SPECT imaging model	Pathology	Sensitivity/ accuracy	Refs.
8	Maraciclatide	^{99m}Tc	Human model	Angiogenesis		[16]
9	3P-RGD2	^{99m}Tc				[16]
10	MSAP-RGD	^{111}In				[1]
11	His-annexin A5 C2AcH-	$^{99m}Tc(CO)3$		Apoptosis		[2]
12	(Me) FGCDEVD	^{99m}Tc				[16]
13	DTPA-Ac-TZ14011	^{111}In		Chemokine receptor 3 expression		[1]
14	AMD3100	^{99m}Tc				[1]
15	DTPA-Fab-PEG24-EGF	^{111}In		Epidermal growth factor receptor		[1]
16	Etarfolatide	^{99m}Tc		Folate receptor		[1]
17	DOTA-folate	^{111}In				[1]
18	MIP1404	^{99m}Tc		Prostate-specific membrane antigen		[1]
19	DPA-alendronate	$^{99m}Tc(CO)3$		Bone imaging		[1]
20	human umbilical tissue-derived cells	^{111}In	Mice model	Cerebral ischemia		[17]
21	^{99m}Tc-pHLIP		Mice model	Lewis lung carcinoma (LLC), lymph node carcinoma of the prostate (LNCaP) and prostate adenocarcinoma	adequate imageability and correlation with tumor extracellular acidity	[18]
22	^{99m}Tc-HHK		Rat model	Tumor microenvironment	High specificity	[18]
23	nanobody (Nb cl1) against CD206 radiolabeled	^{99m}Tc	Mice model	Macrophages in tumor		[18]
24	^{99m}Tc-PyDA		Mice model	In vivo hypoxia targeting	Selective uptake	[18]
25	^{99m}Tc-meropenem			Tumor hypoxia tissue		[18]
26	^{99m}Tc-nitroimidazole		Mice	Differentiate from inflamed and infected tissues		[18]
27	^{99m}Tc-SD32			Breast tumor cells		[18]

Table 9.
SPECT-radiopharmaceuticals using Tc-99m and In-111 for follow-up imaging.

Sr no.	Labeled compound	Labeled radioisotope	SPECT imaging model	Pathology	Sensitivity/ accuracy/ efficiency	Refs.
1.	HMPAO	^{99m}Tc	Human model	Painful prosthetic hip	39% (SD 12%)	[20]
2.	Tropolonate	^{111}In	Human model	Painful prosthetic hip	63% (SD 14%)	[20]
3.	EDDA/HYNIC-TOC	^{99m}Tc	Human model	Cancer diagnosis	High tumor to organ ratio	[21]
4.	P829 peptide	^{99m}Tc	Human model	Neuroendocrine tumors	91%	[22]
5.	Pentetreotide	^{111}In	Human model	Neuroendocrine tumors	65%	[22]
6.	labeled leukocyte	^{111}In	Human model	Osteomyelitis	91%	[23]
7.	HYNIC-TOC	^{99m}Tc	Human model	Metastatic neuroendocrine tumors	Sensitivity 87%	[10]
8.	HYNIC-OC	^{99m}Tc	Human model	Tumor	0.70 ± 0.13%ID/g	[24]
9.	HYNIC-TOC	^{99m}Tc	Human model	Malignancies	3.85 ± 1.0	[24]
10.	HYNIC-TATE	^{99m}Tc	Human model	Tumor	3.99 ± 0.58%ID/g	[24]
11.	DTPA-OC	^{111}In	Human model	Tumor	0.99 ± 0.08%ID/g	[24]
12.	DOTA-TATE	^{111}In	Human model	Tumor	4.12 ± 0.74%ID/g	[24]
13.	Depreotide	^{99m}Tc	Human model	Lung cancer	Immuno-histochemical correlations 98%	[25–28]
14.	DTPA	^{99m}Tc	Human model	Graves' disease	Specificity 89%	[29]
15.	HDP	^{99m}Tc	Human model	Bone imaging		[30]
16.	Tetrofosmin	^{99m}Tc	Human model	Glioblastoma multiforme	L/N ratio of 4.7	[31]
17.	ECD	^{99m}Tc	Human model	Alzheimer's patients		[32]
18.	MAA	^{99m}Tc	Human model	Liver perfusion imaging	100%	[33–35]
19.	Mebrofenin	^{99m}Tc	Human model	Hepatobiliary Scintigraphy		[36]
20.	HSA-DTPA	^{99m}Tc	Human model	Gastrointestinal bleeding	70%	[34]
21.	GHA	^{99m}Tc	Human model	Brain-scanning	85%	[37]
22.	MDP	^{99m}Tc	Human model	Cerebral infarction		[38]
23.	DMSA	^{99m}Tc	Human model	Acute pyelonephritis		[39]

Sr no.	Labeled compound	Labeled radioisotope	SPECT imaging model	Pathology	Sensitivity/ accuracy/ efficiency	Refs.
24.	Pyrophosphate	^{99m}Tc	Human model	Amyloidoses	97%	[40]
25.	Sulfur Nanocolloid	^{99m}Tc	Human model	Lymphatic drainage from prostate	3.9–5.2 mSv/MBq	[41]
26.	Oxine-labeled leukocytes	^{111}In	Human model	Liver cysts	87.5%	
27.	HMPAO-labeled leukocyte	Tc-99m	Human model	Abscess		[42]
28.	MAA-and HAS Microspheres	^{99m}Tc	Human model	Liver-lung shunt		[35]
29.	HSA-DTPA	^{99m}Tc	Human model	Gastrointestinal bleeding	100%	[34]
30.	Labeled bone marrow mesenchymal stem cells	^{111}In	Human model	Acute brain trauma model		[43]
31.	Oxine	^{111}In	Human model	Diagnostic imaging	80%	[42]
32.	HMPAO	^{99m}Tc	Human model	Diagnostic imaging	88%	[42]
33.	Sulfur Nanocolloid	^{99m}Tc	Human model	Mapping of lymphatic drainage from the prostate		[41]
34.	HMPAO-labeled leukocyte	^{99m}Tc	Human model	Prosthetic joint infections	91%	[5]
35.	Labeled chimeric monoclonal antibody Nd2	^{111}In	Human model	Pancreatic cancer	100%	[44]
36.	Labeled GnRH-I tracer	^{111}In	Human model	Tumor imaging	Efficiency $11.8 \pm 1.9\%$	[45]
37.	Oxine labeled mesenchymal stem cells	^{111}In	Human model	Cirrhosis		[46]
38.	TRODAT-1	^{99m}Tc	Human model	Parkinson disease	Target the pre-synaptic dopamine transporter (DAT)	[47]
39.	Depreotide	^{99m}Tc	Human model	Lung cancer and other pulmonary malignancies	96.6%	[4]
40.	Prostascint	^{99m}Tc	Human model	Prostate cancer	Approved	[4]
41.	Zevalin	^{111}In	Human model	Diagnosis of non-Hodgkin's lymphoma	Approved for use	[4]
42.	CEA scan	^{99m}Tc	Human model	Colon cancer	Approved	[4]
	Octreo Scan	^{111}In	Human model	Neuroendocrine tumors		[4]
43.	Depreotide	^{99m}Tc	Human model	Lung cancer		[4]

Sr no.	Labeled compound	Labeled radioisotope	SPECT imaging model	Pathology	Sensitivity/ accuracy/ efficiency	Refs.
44.	Annexin-V	^{99m}Tc	Human model	Acute myocardial infarction and chemotherapy response monitoring		[4]
45.	Neuroligands	^{99m}Tc	Human model	Neuropsychiatric patients		[4]
46.	EC-MN	^{99m}Tc	Human model	Hypoxia		[4]

Table 10.
Clinical trials study of different SPECT radiopharmaceuticals.

A number of SPECT-radiopharmaceuticals are being used in clinical trials which are producing very fruitful results for the diagnosis of different types of cancers and infections in human beings (**Table 10**). These radiolabeled compounds help doctors obtain useful and precise information at a very early stage of the disease to identify the extent of problem and to take timely decisions about the treatment strategies.

Future prospect

There is a need to develop more accurate, sensitive, precise, and reliable SPECT-radiopharmaceuticals to identify the malignant infections and tumors at an early stage in order to overcome the infectious diseases and cancer all over the world. If cancer is diagnosed at an early stage, it would be easier to plan the exact treatment strategy ahead of time. Considerable advancements have been made during last decades in SPECT-radiopharmaceuticals that may take the place of instrumental imaging techniques and therapeutic strategies. In combination with existing technologies, NMT may help a lot in the diagnostic and therapeutic advancement of clinical detection methods.

Author details

Syed Ali Raza Naqvi[1]* and Muhammad Babar Imran[2]

1 Department of Chemistry, Government College University, Faisalabad, Pakistan

2 Punjab Institute of Nuclear Medicine (PINM), Faisalabad, Pakistan

*Address all correspondence to: draliraza@gcuf.edu.pk

IntechOpen

© 2020 The Author(s). Licensee IntechOpen. This chapter is distributed under the terms of the Creative Commons Attribution License (http://creativecommons.org/licenses/by/3.0), which permits unrestricted use, distribution, and reproduction in any medium, provided the original work is properly cited. (cc) BY

References

[1] Payolla FB et al. Radiopharmaceuticals for diagnosis in nuclear medicine: A short review. Eclética Química Journal. 2019;**44**:11-19

[2] Navalkissoor S et al. Single-photon emission computed tomography–computed tomography in imaging infection. Nuclear Medicine Communications. 2013;**34**:283-290

[3] Sathekge M et al. Molecular imaging in musculoskeletal infections with (99m)Tc-UBI 29-41 SPECT/CT. Annals of Nuclear Medicine. 2018;**32**(1):54-59

[4] Imam SK. Molecular nuclear imaging: The radiopharmaceuticals (review). Cancer Biotherapy & Radiopharmaceuticals. 2005;**20**(2): 163-172

[5] Kim HO et al. Usefulness of adding SPECT/CT to 99mTc-hexamethylpropylene amine oxime (HMPAO)-labeled leukocyte imaging for diagnosing prosthetic joint infections. Journal of Computer Assisted Tomography. 2014;**38**(2):313-319

[6] Su H-C et al. Evaluation of 99mTc-labeled PSMA-SPECT/CT imaging in prostate cancer patients who have undergone biochemical relapse. Asian Journal of Andrology. 2017;**19**(3): 267-271

[7] England CG et al. Molecular imaging of pancreatic cancer with antibodies. Molecular Pharmaceutics. 2016;**13**(1): 8-24

[8] Abikhzer G, Keidar Z. SPECT/CT and tumour imaging. European Journal of Nuclear Medicine and Molecular Imaging. 2013;**41**(Suppl 1):S67-S80

[9] Miao Y, Benwell K, Quinn TP. 99mTc- and 111In-labeled alpha-melanocyte-stimulating hormone peptides as imaging probes for primary and pulmonary metastatic melanoma detection. Journal of Nuclear Medicine. 2007;**48**(1):73-80

[10] Artiko V et al. The clinical value of scintigraphy of neuroendocrine tumors using (99m)Tc-HYNIC-TOC. Journal of BUON. 2012;**17**(3):537-542

[11] Gabriel M et al. An intrapatient comparison of 99mTc-EDDA/HYNIC-TOC with 111In-DTPA-octreotide for diagnosis of somatostatin receptor-expressing tumors. Journal of Nuclear Medicine. 2003;**44**(5):708-716

[12] Cusso L et al. Combination of single-photon emission computed tomography and magnetic resonance imaging to track 111in-oxine-labeled human mesenchymal stem cells in neuroblastoma-bearing mice. Molecular Imaging. 2014;**13**

[13] Dar U et al. In house development of (99m)Tc-rhenium sulfide colloidal nanoparticles for sentinel lymph node detection. Pakistan Journal of Pharmaceutical Sciences. 2013;**26**: 367-373

[14] Sadeghi S et al. Development of (111)In-labeled porphyrins for SPECT imaging. Asia Oceania Journal of Nuclear Medicine & Biology. 2014;**2**(2): 95-103

[15] Harris TD et al. Structure-activity relationships of 111In- and 99mTc-labeled quinolin-4-one peptidomimetics as ligands for the vitronectin receptor: Potential tumor imaging agents. Bioconjugate Chemistry. 2006;**17**(5): 1294-1313

[16] Gnanasegaran G, Ballinger JR. Molecular imaging agents for SPECT (and SPECT/CT). European Journal of Nuclear Medicine and Molecular Imaging. 2014;**41**(Suppl 1):S26-S35

[17] Arbab AS et al. Tracking of In-111-labeled human umbilical tissue-derived cells (hUTC) in a rat model of cerebral ischemia using SPECT imaging. BMC Medical Imaging. 2012;**12**(1):33

[18] Abadjian MZ, Edwards WB, Anderson CJ. Imaging the tumor microenvironment. Advances in Experimental Medicine and Biology. 2017;**1036**:229-257

[19] Schmitt A et al. Differences in biodistribution between 99mTc-depreotide, 111In-DTPA-octreotide, and 177Lu-DOTA-Tyr3-octreotate in a small cell lung cancer animal model. Cancer Biotherapy & Radiopharmaceuticals. 2005;**20**(2):231-236

[20] Aktolun C et al. Technetium-99m and indium-111 double labelling of granulocytes for kinetic and clinical studies. European Journal of Nuclear Medicine. 1995;**22**(4):330-334

[21] Decristoforo C et al. 99mTc-EDDA/HYNIC-TOC: A new 99mTc-labelled radiopharmaceutical for imaging somatostatin receptor-positive tumours; first clinical results and intra-patient comparison with 111In-labelled octreotide derivatives. European Journal of Nuclear Medicine. 2000;**27**(9):1318-1325

[22] Lebtahi R et al. Detection of neuroendocrine tumors: 99mTc-P829 scintigraphy compared with 111In-pentetreotide scintigraphy. Journal of Nuclear Medicine. 2002;**43**(7):889-895

[23] Palestro CJ et al. Osteomyelitis: Diagnosis with (99m)Tc-labeled antigranulocyte antibodies compared with diagnosis with (111)In-labeled leukocytes—initial experience. Radiology. 2002;**223**(3):758-764

[24] Storch D et al. Evaluation of [99mTc/EDDA/HYNIC0]octreotide derivatives compared with [111In-DOTA0,Tyr3, Thr8]octreotide and [111In-DTPA0]octreotide: Does tumor or pancreas uptake correlate with the rate of internalization? Journal of Nuclear Medicine. 2005;**46**(9):1561-1569

[25] Herlin G et al. Quantitative assessment of 99mTc-depreotide uptake in patients with non-small-cell lung cancer: Immunohistochemical correlations. Acta Radiologica. 2009;**50**(8):902-908

[26] Axelsson R et al. Role of scintigraphy with technetium-99m depreotide in the diagnosis and management of patients with suspected lung cancer. Acta Radiologica. 2008;**49**(3):295-302

[27] Shih W-J et al. 99mTc-depreotide chest SPECT demonstrates pulmonary metastases from renal cell carcinoma. Journal of Nuclear Medicine Technology. 2004;**32**(1):19-21

[28] Harders SW et al. Limited value of 99mTc depreotide single photon emission CT compared with CT for the evaluation of pulmonary lesions. The British Journal of Radiology. 2012;**85**(1015):e307-e313

[29] Szumowski P et al. Efficacy of (99m)Tc-DTPA SPECT/CT in diagnosing orbitopathy in graves' disease. BMC Endocrine Disorders. 2019;**19**(1):10-10

[30] Hirschmann MT et al. Assessment of loading history of compartments in the knee using bone SPECT/CT: A study combining alignment and 99mTc-HDP tracer uptake/distribution patterns. Journal of Orthopaedic Research. 2013;**31**(2):268-274

[31] Alexiou GA et al. The value of 99mTc-tetrofosmin brain SPECT in predicting survival in patients with glioblastoma multiforme. Journal of Nuclear Medicine. 2010;**51**(12):1923-1926

[32] Merhof D et al. Optimized data preprocessing for multivariate analysis applied to 99mTc-ECD SPECT data sets of Alzheimer's patients and asymptomatic controls. Journal of Cerebral Blood Flow and Metabolism: Official Journal of the International Society of Cerebral Blood Flow and Metabolism. 2011;**31**(1):371-383

[33] Ahmadzadehfar H et al. The significance of 99mTc-MAA SPECT/CT liver perfusion imaging in treatment planning for 90Y-microsphere selective internal radiation treatment. Journal of Nuclear Medicine. 2010;**51**(8):1206-1212

[34] Kotani K et al. Diagnostic ability of 99mTc-HSA-DTPA scintigraphy in combination with SPECT/CT for gastrointestinal bleeding. Abdominal Imaging. 2014;**39**(4):677-684

[35] Grosser OS et al. Pharmacokinetics of 99mTc-MAA- and 99mTc-HSA-microspheres used in preradioembolization dosimetry: Influence on the liver–lung shunt. Journal of Nuclear Medicine. 2016; **57**(6):925-927

[36] de Graaf W et al. 99mTc-mebrofenin hepatobiliary scintigraphy with SPECT for the assessment of hepatic function and liver functional volume before partial hepatectomy. Journal of Nuclear Medicine. 2010; **51**(2):229-236

[37] Santra A, Kumar R, Sharma P. Use of 99m-technetium-glucoheptonate as a tracer for brain tumor imaging: An overview of its strengths and pitfalls. Indian Journal of Nuclear Medicine: IJNM: The Official Journal of the Society of Nuclear Medicine, India. 2015;**30**(1):1-8

[38] Guo J et al. Cerebral infarction on 99mTc-MDP SPECT/CT imaging. Clinical Nuclear Medicine. 2013;**38**:925-927

[39] Yoo JM et al. Diagnosing acute pyelonephritis with CT, 99mTc-DMSA SPECT, and Doppler ultrasound: A comparative study. Korean Journal of Urology. 2010;**51**(4):260-265

[40] Bokhari S et al. ^{99m}Tc-pyrophosphate scintigraphy for differentiating light-chain cardiac amyloidosis from the transthyretin-related familial and senile cardiac amyloidoses. Circulation. Cardiovascular Imaging. 2013;**6**(2):195-201

[41] Seo Y et al. Mapping of lymphatic drainage from the prostate using filtered 99mTc-sulfur nanocolloid and SPECT/CT. Journal of Nuclear Medicine. 2011; **52**(7):1068-1072

[42] Djekidel M, Brown RKJ, Piert M. Benefits of hybrid SPECT/CT for 111In-oxine- and Tc-99m-hexamethylpropylene amine oxime-labeled leukocyte imaging. Clinical Nuclear Medicine. 2011;**36**(7):e50-e56

[43] Yoon JK et al. In vivo tracking of 111In-labeled bone marrow mesenchymal stem cells in acute brain trauma model. Nuclear Medicine and Biology. 2010;**37**(3):381-388

[44] Sawada T et al. Preoperative clinical radioimmunodetection of pancreatic cancer by 111In-labeled chimeric monoclonal antibody Nd2. Japanese Journal of Cancer Research. 1999; **90**(10):1179-1186

[45] Zoghi M et al. Evaluation of 111In-labeled GnRH-I tracer for SPECT tumor imaging. Radiochemistry. 2019;**61**(2): 226-232

[46] Gholamrezanezhad A et al. In vivo tracking of 111In-oxine labeled mesenchymal stem cells following infusion in patients with advanced cirrhosis. Nuclear Medicine and Biology. 2011;**38**(7):961-967

[47] Zhu L, Ploessl K, Kung HF. PET/SPECT imaging agents for neurodegenerative diseases. Chemical Society Reviews. 2014;**43**(19):6683-6691

Chapter 2

Gallium-68: Radiolabeling of Radiopharmaceuticals for PET Imaging - A Lot to Consider

Michael Meisenheimer, Yury Saenko and Elisabeth Eppard

Abstract

Gallium-68 was applied for positron emission tomography (PET) imaging already in the early beginnings of PET imaging. Today, with the introduction of PSMA-targeting tracers (e.g. PSMA-11, PSMA-617, and PSMA-I&T), the number of clinical applications of ^{68}Ga-radiopharmaceuticals for diagnostic imaging has grown considerably. This development was initiated and supported already in the mid-2000s by the commercial availability of ^{68}Ge/^{68}Ga generators designed for clinical usage. This progression was accompanied by the development of several purification methods to generator eluate as well as sophisticated ^{68}Ga-radiopharmaceuticals. Due to the ^{68}Ga-rush, the need for implementation of gallium-68 (depending on production route) and its certain tracers into the pharmacopeia increased. Based on the specifications given by the pharmacopeia, interest focused on the development of automated synthesis systems, ^{99m}Tc-analog kits with regard to patient as well as operator safety.

Keywords: gallium-68, radiopharmaceuticals, production, quality control, clinical use

1. Introduction

In recent years, ^{68}Ga-radiopharmaceuticals gained more and more attention due to their steadily growing clinical application. Facilitated is this development by increasing interest in the application of its "theranostic twin" lutetium-177. Combining both, gallium-68 and lutetium-177, enables diagnostic molecular imaging followed by personalized treatment based on the diagnostic scan [1].

This concept is well established for treatment of neuroendocrine tumors (NETs) using peptide receptor radionuclide therapy (PRRT). This approach allows the targeted treatment of inoperable or metastatic NETs already proven in multiple clinical trials employing radiolabeled somatostatin analogs [2–9]. Based on the data received, the U.S. Food and Drug Administration (FDA) recently approved ^{177}Lu-labeled DOTA-TATE for PRRT treatment. However, not only for NETs, but also for other types of cancer (e.g. prostate cancer (PC)), lutetium-177 is of interest, reflected in numerous clinical trials registered at https://clinicaltrials.gov (keyword: lutetium-177; 87 trials; 12/9/2019). Even more trials are enrolled for its diagnostic counterpart gallium-68 (keyword: gallium-68; 268 trials; 12/9/2019). While only a handful clinical trials were conducted before 2012 for both radionuclides (gallium-68, 12 trials between 1991 and 2011; lutetium-177, 16 trials between 1996 and 2011) both have increasingly found application in clinical routine reflected in the rapidly increasing amount of enrolled phase 1–3 studies.

Although, gallium-68 was already proposed for medical use by Gleason [10] its way to clinical application was not possible without the advancement of the primary generator design. Providing $[^{68}Ga]GaCl_3$ and containing only trace levels of the long-living mother radionuclide germanium-68 regarding ^{68}Ga-activity, the commercially availability of generator simplified research and motivated developments with a view to a broad routine application. The launch of this new type of ^{68}Ga-generator together with decades of research in chelation chemistry and drug discovery resulted in the design of ^{68}Ga-radiopharmaceuticals of high affinity/selectivity for their biological targets [11–13].

The advantages of the generator availability and the easy one-step chelation chemistry ensured the relatively fast and broad application of the ^{68}Ga-radiopharmaceuticals even in smaller institutions. However, exactly these advantages lead to problems in the supply today and require new developments in order to meet the growing demands.

2. Application: why choosing a radiometal?

What is the advantage of radiometals for an application in nuclear medicine? With carbon-11 and mostly fluor-18, two radionuclides for positron emission tomography (PET) are available, which can be used for radiolabeling without appreciably altering the biological properties of the compounds in addition to their favorable decay characteristics. However, the disadvantage of radiometals, the need for a chelator is also their advantage over fluor-18 and carbon-11.

Due to this, radiolabeling with radiometals is very easy, can be conducted in aqueous solution and with the right choice of chelator possible under mild conditions. That enables radiolabeling of temperature or organic solvent sensitive compounds (e.g. antibodies). Additionally, the choice of chelator provides the possibility of radiolabeling one compound with different radiometals. Thus,

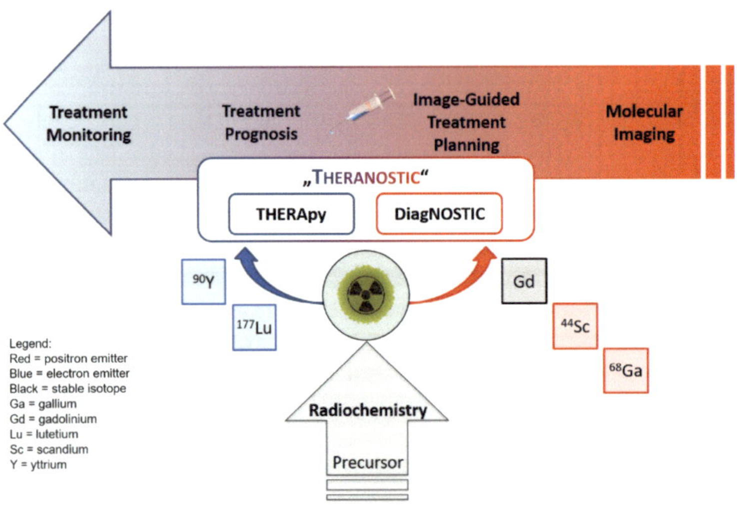

Figure 1.
Depiction of the theranostic concept: utilizing one compound for a variety of applications in patient-centered care radiolabeled with different radionuclide.

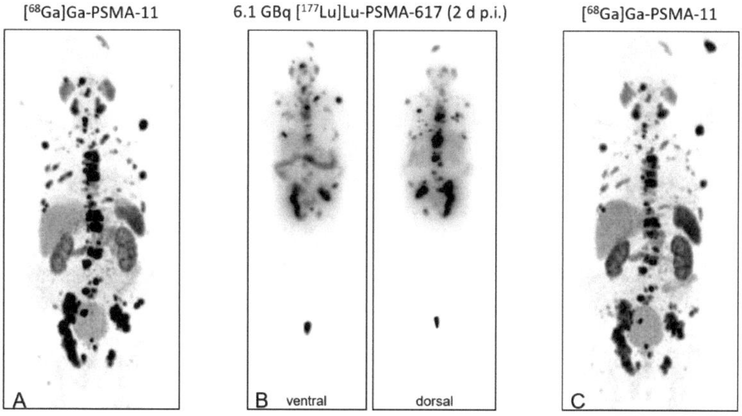

Figure 2.
PET-images (A; C) and SPECT-images (B) of a patient with metastatic castrate-resistant prostate cancer (mCRPC) undergoing therapy with [^{177}Lu]Lu-PSMA-617 with pre- and posttherapeutic ^{68}Ga-PET-imaging using the diagnostic counterpart [^{68}Ga]Ga-PSMA-11.

widespread application (PET, single photon emission computed tomography (SPECT), magnet resonance tomography (MRT) and therapy) of the compound only by exchange of the radiometal with minimum changes in biological behavior is possible. This facilitates patient-centered care from diagnosis via molecular imaging, over treatment planning, prognosis and monitoring utilizing one compound (**Figure 1**).

Advantages in favor of gallium-68 compared with other appropriate radiometals are its favorable decay characteristics, its (commercial) availability and the possible combination with lutetium-177 as theranostic pair (**Figure 2**). Also gallium-68 possibly provides patient care in places where cyclotron-produced fluor-18 is not obtainable.

3. Current applications of ^{68}Ga-radiopharmaceuticals

Currently gallium-68 is most widely used in the diagnosis of prostate cancer in the form of [^{68}Ga]Ga-PSMA-11, respectively. [^{68}Ga]Ga-PSMA-617 together with [^{177}Lu]Lu-DOTA-PSMA-617 forms a theranostic couple, which is very well suited for the diagnosis or treatment of prostate cancer as the ^{68}Ga/^{177}Lu-radiolabelled tracers show a very similar biological behavior. Due to similarities in chemical behavior, identical (in case of PSMA-617) precursors can be radiolabelled using the same or similar equipment, synthesis and quality control methods [14].

The second, but longest known and best evaluated, ^{68}Ga theranostic pair is used for neuroendocrine tumors in combination with various somatostatin analogs. The three most widely used analogs of somatostatin with gallium-68 are [^{68}Ga]Ga-DOTA-TOC, [^{68}Ga]Ga-DOTA-TATE, [^{68}Ga]Ga-DOTA-LAN or [^{68}Ga]Ga-DOTA-NOC [15]. As a therapeutic counterpart, yttrium-90 and lutetium-177 are used.

Besides these two main applications of gallium-68, a variety of studies work on the extension of the application scope.

For imaging of insulinoma pancreatic islets, several versions of ^{68}Ga-radiopharmaceuticals based on Exendin-4, a glucagon-like protein-1 receptor agonist, exist and it was demonstrated that [^{68}Ga]Ga-DOTA-exendin-4 localizes insulinoma significantly better than ^{111}In-radiolabelled radiopharmaceuticals [16].

Integrin αvβ3 and gastrin-releasing peptide receptor (GRPR) are usually overexpressed in human breast cancer, prostate cancer, breast cancer, colorectal cancer, pancreatic cancer, glioma, lung cancer, ovarian cancers, endometrial cancers, renal cell cancer and gastrointestinal stromal tumors. An amphibian homolog of the mammalian gastrin-releasing peptide bombesin was intensively investigated, also radiolabelled with gallium-68, for imaging of GRPR. For integrin $\alpha v\beta 3$, specific imaging probes usually use the peptide arginine-glycine-aspartic acid (RGD). For imagine of GRPR, several radiopharmaceuticals based on gallium-68 were proposed, in particular [^{68}Ga]Ga-BBN-RGD for breast cancer imagine [17], [^{68}Ga]Ga-NOTA-Aca-BBN for glioma imagine [18], [^{68}Ga]-NOTA-DUPA-RM26 for prostate cancer imagine.

Another promising area of application of ^{68}Ga-based radiopharmaceuticals is the labeling of human epidermal growth factor receptor family (HER2) [19] and carcinoembryonic antigen (CEA) [20].

Even though gallium-68 is a very convenient radionuclide for use in radiopharmacy, it is widespread in radiopharmaceuticals in comparison with other diagnostic isotopes. But usability and the commercially availability of generator simplified research and motivated developments with a view to a broad routine application.

4. Radiometals: special needs?

Radiolabeling with radiometals is in some ways challenging. Due to the very low amount of substance, other metals present in the reaction mixture can be serious problem and noticeably effect the radiolabeling. These metallic impurities can compete with gallium-68 for the chelating function of the precursor and are compared with gallium-68 (1 GBq equals to 9.73×10^{-12} mol) even when present at low levels (<ppm) clearly in excess number. They are result of external influences (e.g. production of starting materials) or are an intrinsic generator property (e.g. matrix; decay product). To avoid additional or larger impurities than necessary, the following is recommended by the IAEA [21]:

- Use plastic disposables/contact materials
- Avoid contact with metals of your working equipment during preparation of reagents (e.g. pipettes, spatulas, vials, etc.)
- Protect your working materials from direct contact with metals (e.g. surfaces, etc.)
- Use chemicals and water with lowest metal content as possible (e.g. ultra-pure grade)
- Do not use standard laboratory glassware (e.g. beakers, etc.)
- Consider coating of your fume hood.

5. Gallium-68: a brief profile

Gallium is located in group 13 in the 4th period. It has 31 known isotopes and 11 metastable isomers including the two natural occurring stable isotopes gallium-69 (60.11%) and gallium-71 (39.89%). Two gallium isotopes are applied in nuclear medicine for PET-imaging: gallium-67, which has the longest half-life ($T_{1/2}$ = 3.26 d) of the instable ^{68}Ga-isotopes, and gallium-68 ($T_{1/2}$ = 67.71 min).

Positron emitter	Half-life	$\widetilde{E}_{\beta}$	$E_{\beta, max}$
		[MeV]	
Gallium-68	67.71 min	0.829	1.899
Flourine-18	109.77 min	0.250	0.634

Table 1.
Comparison of mean ($\widetilde{E}_{\beta}$) and maximum ($E_{\beta, max}$) positron energies of gallium-68 and fluorine-18 [24].

Ga(III) is a hard Lewis acid forming complexes coordinating four, five or six ligands. The most stable complexes are the last-mentioned with a octahedral coordination sphere in which oxygen, nitrogen and sulfur donor atoms form coordination bonds with Ga(III). To ensure the complex formation thorough pH, control is required to ensure deprotonation of the electron donor and to protect Ga(III) from forming $Ga(OH)_3$ precipitating at pH 3–7 [22].

Gallium-68 is a positron emitter that decays with a half-life of 67.71 min and 89% positron branching to stable zinc-68. The transition is accompanied by low-abundant photon emission (1077 keV, 3.22%) [23]. **Table 1** shows the mean and maximum energies of the positrons emitted in comparison to fluorine-18.

6. Availability: sources of gallium-68

6.1 Traditional: $^{68}Ge/^{68}Ga$-generator

One of the reasons of the emerging application of gallium-68 in nuclear medicine is its cyclotron-independency and availability via radionuclide generator. Since the application of gallium-68 was a long time limited to research, advancements in generator design facilitated research on new ^{68}Ga-radiopharmaceuticals as well as clinical use of the known.

Physical basis for radionuclide generators is the existence of the radioactive equilibria. The differentiation between radionuclide generations is based on the half-lives of the parent (1) and its daughter (2). Depending on the ratio between the two half-lives, three principal cases can be distinguished:

1. Transient equilibrium. Longer living parent but not more than factor 100: $T_{1/2, 2} < T_{1/2,1} < 100$.

2. Secular equilibrium. Much longer living parent: $T_{1/2, 2} << T_{1/2,1}$.

3. No equilibrium. Shorter living parent.

The basis for the $^{68}Ge/^{68}Ga$-generator is the secular equilibrium between the parent radionuclide germanium-68 and its daughter gallium-68. Germanium-68 decays with $T_{1/2}$ = 270.95 days via electron capture to gallium-68. This transition is subsequently followed by decay of gallium-68 to stable zinc-68. At equilibrium, the quantity of gallium-68 produced is equal to the quantity of gallium-68 decaying, while the parent activity does not significantly decrease over many half-lives of the daughter. The theoretical maximum activity or equilibrium state for a certain generator system can be obtained at the time t (**Figure 3**):

$$t = \frac{1}{\lambda_2 - \lambda_1} ln \frac{\lambda_2}{\lambda_1} \quad (1)$$

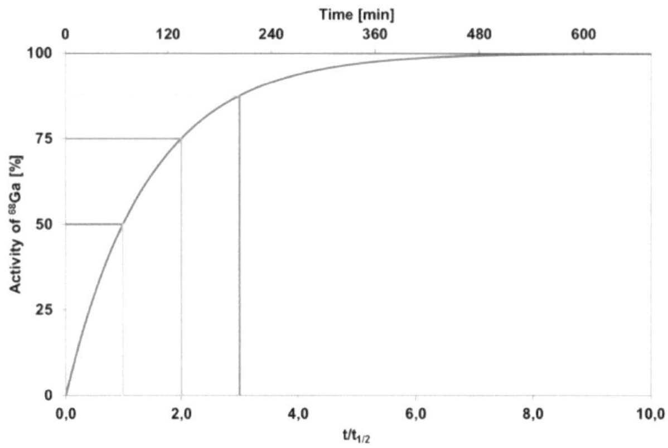

Figure 3.
Build-up kinetics of gallium-68 on the generator column after initial elution.

For the $^{68}Ge/^{68}Ga$ system, equilibrium is reached after 14.1 h, representing maximum obtainable activity. Even if idle times of 12.5 half-lives are necessary to obtain maximum activities, the generators can be used more frequently. Within two half-lives of gallium-68 already 75% of the maximum value is build-up and could be used.

The $^{68}Ge/^{68}Ga$-generator system introduced in the 1960s by Gleason [10] underwent a lot of changes until today. From the first gallium cow providing gallium-68 after liquid–liquid extraction [10], nowadays the generators, based on a solid matrix (inorganic or organic) providing "ionic" $^{68}Ga^{3+}$ eluates. The first commercially available generator of this type was developed by Cyclotron Ltd., Obninsk, Russian Federation [25] eluting gallium-68 with 0.1 M HCl with initial elution yields of ~80% and ^{68}Ge breakthrough of 0.001% [26]. Since the introduction of this generator in 1996 [26], a lot has happened on the market. Today several manufacturers produce $^{68}Ge/^{68}Ga$-generators, including ones with GMP grade (e.g. Isotopen Technologien Garching (ITG)) or with approval (e.g. GalliPharm® Eckert & Ziegler in the EU with marketing authorization, in the USA with type II drug master file (DMF) on file with FDA).

Even though these generators represent considerable improvements in ^{68}Ga-production, there are still some obstacles to direct radiolabeling with gallium-68. Beside the low radioactive and high [H^+] concentration and ^{68}Ge breakthrough, especially the presence of other trivalent metal ions is an inconvenience. As 1 GBq gallium-68 is equal to 9.73 pmol (9.73×10^{-12} mol), these metallic impurities, even present at low levels (<ppm), can be a serious problem as they can compete with gallium-68 for the chelating function of the precursor. In addition to the IAEA recommendations on externally introduced metallic contaminations [21], several procedures are available to reduce those metallic impurities, either intrinsic or externally introduced. These post-elution purification methods, so called post-processing's, aim to improve the radioactive and [H^+] concentration and the radionuclidic as well as chemical purity of the ^{68}Ga-eluate. Beside fractionation of the eluate [11], anion-exchange (AEX) [13], cation-exchange (CEX) [27–29] and a combination thereof [30, 31] found to be suitable but only for fractionation but also are commercially used for cation-exchange.

6.2 Work in progress: cyclotron

Although $^{68}Ge/^{68}Ga$-generators represent a convenient possibility for persistent patient care with ^{68}Ga-radiopharmaceuticals, their ^{68}Ga-activity available for radiolabeling underlies several restrictions resulting from generator design and physics. In conjunction with the sharp increase in demand in recent years, alternative production routes, preferably realizable with existing medical cyclotrons, moved into the focus.

Small to medium energy medical cyclotrons are suitable for ^{68}Ga-production via the ^{68}Zn(p,n)^{68}Ga reaction using either a solid or a liquid target. Among the possible nuclear reactions [32, 33], it is the most reasonable leading to large production yields. For optimal results, the starting material zinc-68 as well as the proton energy needs to be selected with care to reduce co-production of long-living radioisotopes of gallium. Nevertheless, co-production of gallium-66 and gallium-67 is unavoidable due to the starting material and the excitation function of the ^{68}Zn(p,2n)^{67}Ga reaction [32, 33]. This has to be taken into account when producing gallium-68 via cyclotron for radiopharmaceutical application as both radioisotopes cannot be separated from the desired gallium-68.

For production of gallium-68 via cyclotron, either a solid or a liquid target can be used. For both target types, a lot of options exist leading to a several considerations to be made. Solid targets, for example, can be pressed, electroplated, foil or fused, all types having their advantages and disadvantages which are not mentioned here. In a first instance, the choice of target will mostly be done due to the actual conditions of the site. An existing production site for ^{18}F-compounds which want to implement gallium-68 would probably choose the liquid target route, as the preconditions for a solid target (target holder, cooling, target transfer and target processing) are expensive and likely not available. Compared with that, the liquid target is a quick and inexpensive option to obtain gallium-68 when a generator is not reasonable. A detailed overview about all possible alternatives and their advantages/disadvantages is given by the IAEA [21].

After irradiation, the gallium-68 needs to be purified from target material either if a solid or liquid target was used. The quantity of zinc necessary for the target need to be removed as it and all other metal impurities may perturb the radiolabeling reaction of gallium-68. Intense research on this topic lead to several purification methods based on solvent extraction [34, 35], precipitation [36] and solid phase separation [37–44] and suitable for automation.

Solid-phase extraction using a cation exchange resin or hydroxamate resin is most appropriate for an effective separation of gallium-68 from unwanted metals and can be easily combined with a second resin. This second purification step allows an additional reduction of [H^+] concentration to facilitate further processing of the final product [21]:

- Local conditions (expertise and equipment)
- Separation time (should be as short as possible)
- Acids (concentration and volume)
- Availability of materials
- Robustness of technique
- Ease of automation
- Possibility to recycle zinc-68 from target solution

7. Radiolabeling: complexation chemistry in clinical settings

7.1 Manual

The manual radiolabeling approach is a leftover from times, where gallium-68 was mainly used for research purpose, with lower ^{68}Ga-activities and not in a clinical setting for patient care. It is widely used in research and development of new tracers [11–13, 29, 30, 45–51]. Its main advantage is full control over the complete process (pH, time and temperature) and the possibility to easily access radiolabeling kinetics.

Due to its general setup, this method is not suitable and indented for clinical use. Nevertheless, before the introduction of module systems or the cold kits, it was a long time, the only available method.

In general (**Figure 4**), the first step is the preparation of the reaction mixture by mixing [^{68}Ga]$GaCl_3$ with a suitable buffer in the required pH range and the radiolabeling precursor. Here, the purified cyclotron-produced, generator eluate or post-processed gallium-68 can be used.

Then, the reaction vial is incubated to form the ^{68}Ga-complex. Reaction period and reaction temperature are selected in accordance to the kinetics of the complex formation of gallium with the used chelator.

After the reaction, the reaction mixture can be purified using, for example, solid phase extraction from, for example, free gallium-68 and residual germanium-68 impurities.

In the final step, the ^{68}Ga-radiopharmaceutical is sterile filtrated and formulated in the product vial (**Table 2**).

7.2 Module

With the growing interest for gallium-68 not only for research but also for clinical routine and patient care the need for pharmacopeia compliant preparation of ^{68}Ga-radiopharmaceuticals. This led to promotion of the automation of the traditional manual synthesis from which numerous semi- and fully automated devices have emerged. Today, those systems are designed with respect to Good

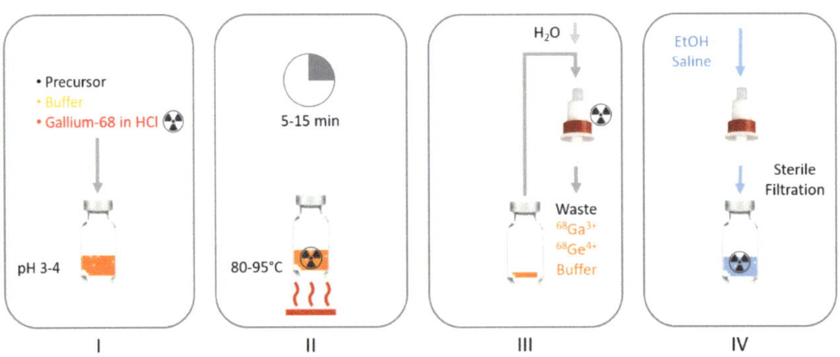

Figure 4.
Schematic description of the ^{68}Ga-radiolabeling procedure (I) preparation of the reaction mixture by adding gallium-68 eluted from a generator or after post-processing to a mixture of a suitable buffer and precursor, (II) incubation of the reaction mixture for a certain time. If elevated temperatures are needed or not depends on the chelator, (III) purification step using solid phase extraction (SPE). For example, the ^{68}Ga-radiopharmaceutical is trapped on a SPE C18-cartridge where it is washed with water to remove free gallium-68, germanium-68 and buffer, (IV) the purified product is finally eluted with diluted ethanol solution and formulated after sterile filtration in the product vial.

Chelator	Radiolabeling conditions
DOTA	37–90°C, 10–30 min, pH 4.0–5.5 [52, 53]
HBED	25°C, 10–20 min, pH 4.0–4.5 [54]

Table 2.
Radiolabeling conditions for gallium-68 for DOTA and HBED.

Manufacturing Practice (GMP) Guidelines provided, for example, by the FDA, EU/EMA, ICH, WHO or others [55]. They use software and methods designed to minimize user interventions and utilize single-use consumables produced under GMP standard.

While the module production requires a fully equipped laboratory and quality control, it reduces radiation exposure of the operator the production process in terms of higher reliability and reduced variability [56–58].

Accordingly, the amount of contaminated waste materials is higher due to the procedure as well the complete quality control. Nevertheless, these systems are suitable for a variety of tracers and in most cases for more radionuclides not only for gallium-68 (e.g. Scintomics GRP series; Eckert & Ziegler Modular-Lab PharmTracer; Trasis AllInOne).

7.3 Kits

Recently, cold kits for radiolabeling entered the scene enable production of ^{68}Ga-radiopharmaceuticals as easy as that of ^{99m}Tc-radiopharmaceuticals. This method allows the reconstitution of the pre-formulated cold kit with no previous post-processing of the eluate or subsequent purification of the final product. They are available in GMP quality and leaves only minimum quality control tests to the final user responsibility to verify the reconstitution procedure.

For example, the European Pharmacopeia (Ph. Eur.) states the marketing authorization (MA) holder of a licensed kit is responsible to ensure compliance of the kit with the requirements of its MA, while the final user carries the responsibility for the quality of the preparation and the handling. If the given instructions are not strictly followed or if one or more components used for the reconstitution do not have MA, it is the responsibility of the final user to demonstrate that the quality of the final preparation is suitable for the intended, use [26].

Therefore, preparation as well as quality control requires at least the equipment according to the instructions provided by the manufacturer. In addition, minimum contaminated waste materials remain. It has to be noted, according to the Ph. Eur. that applies only for licensed kits in combination with the generator mentioned in the instructions from the manufacturer. In contrast, unlicensed kits or a licensed kit used with an unlicensed generator or cyclotron produced gallium-68 also require full quality control according to the monograph. Additionally, local authorities may require more detailed quality control even for licensed kits.

Indeed, these cold kits contain relatively high amounts of precursor and additional filler materials. They still require manual handling and are only commercially available as single-dose kits for radiolabeling PSMA-11 (e.g. illumet™) and DOTA-TOC (e.g. NETSPOT®). In addition, the use of unpurified generator eluates requires very strict specifications for the generators in terms of ^{68}Ge-breakthrough to ensure the quality of the final product. Nevertheless, there is a possibility for small sites to offer ^{68}Ga-radiopharmaceuticals to their patients without great expense.

8. Quality control: pharmaceutical needs and radioactive specialties

Quality defects of pharmaceutical can lead to serious consequences when they are applied. Consequently, the regulatory framework for production and quality control is very strict. In general, one main requirement in the production of pharmaceuticals is a comprehensive, integrated system of quality assurance. Its purpose is the monitoring and documentation of all processes as well as their functionality with respect to the rules of GMP.

Because radiopharmaceuticals are pharmaceutical preparations containing minimum one radionuclide for diagnostic or therapeutic purpose, in principle the same rules apply. Their quality control is intended to ensure that the quality meets the predefined specifications for the radiopharmaceutical. These specifications take into account the radionuclide, the precursor, the preparation process, the formulation and the intended administration route. Due to the nature of the contained radionuclides, not all necessary quality control tests can be performed before release for administration and require retrospective examination. In the available monographs, it is indicated if a test need not to be completed before release of the batch.

In the case of gallium-68, the short half-live and the limited available activities lead to further challenges. Here are sophisticated logistics for preparation and quality control essential.

In general, quality control of ^{68}Ga-radiopharmaceuticals should include the following tests and information [59–61]:

1. *Characters/appearance*. Should discover any visible container defects. The quality of the final product in terms of absence of particular matter [62] and/or turbidity should be ensured as well as its correct appearance. Typically performed by visual inspection.

2. *pH determination*. Should ensure that the pH of the final product is in the necessary range for its purpose. For the final injectable formulation of a radiopharmaceutical, the pH should be closed to the physiologic value of 7.4. With regard to the relatively low volume of radiopharmaceuticals and depending on the injected volume and rate, a wider range (3.5–8.5) is applicable. Contrary to this, the pH of the radionuclide precursor gallium-68 should not exceed 2 to prevent the formation of unwanted ^{68}Ga-colloids.

3. *Radionuclidic identification*. Identification of a radionuclide is generally conducted by determination of its half-life and/the nature and energy of its radiation emitted. For positron emitters like gallium-68 instead of energy and nature of the radiation, the identification is based on a γ-spectrum additional to their half-life determination (e.g. with dose calibrator).

4. *Radiochemical identification.* Identification of the desired radiochemical species via HPLC and/or TLC exploiting different chemical behavior of the different radiochemical species.

5. *Radionuclidic purity*. Due to the contribution or formation of other radionuclides during the production of gallium-68, their amount present in the final radiopharmaceutical must be determined. Depending on the production route of gallium-68, different limits for radionuclidic impurities may apply. The test for those long-living radionuclides need to be performed after complete decay of the sample using γ-spectrometry, representing a test performed after release of the batch.

6. *Radiochemical purity*. Should discover all chemical forms containing the radionuclide and determine their percentage of the total radioactivity of the product. These radiochemical impurities arise from the synthesis method, radiolysis or the radionuclide production and can lower the quality of the final diagnostic examination. Principally be determined by any suitable analytical method but with respect to the short half-life and radiation TLC and HPLC are normally used for quality control of ^{68}Ga-radiopharmaceuticals.

7. *Chemical purity*. The chemical purity refers to the amount of the specified chemical form of a preparation if radioactivity is present or not [61]. Purity assessment is of special importance when diagnostic or therapeutic properties are directly linked to chemistry [63]. Therefore, particular attention is necessary for pharmacologically active impurities as they can affect the diagnostic value of the examination. The chemical purity of ^{68}Ga-radiopharmaceuticals is normally ascertained with TLC and/or HPLC.

8. *Residual solvents*. Ph. Eur. as well as US pharmacopeia defines residual solvents as organic volatile chemicals used in the manufacture of drug substances/active substances, excipients or in the preparation of medicinal products (Eur. Ph. 5.4.; USP 467). As they represent a risk of health, they should be determined. Determination can be performed using gas chromatography (GC)

It has to be noted that the texts about residual solvents not cover solvents added by purpose or solvates. For those other limits and regulations may apply.

9. *Microbiological contamination*. Parenteral administered radiopharmaceuticals need to be compliant in terms of bacterial endotoxins or pyrogens as well as sterility

Bacterial endotoxins are known to cause a wide spectrum of nonspecific pathophysiological reactions (fever, changes in white blood cell counts, hypotension, disseminated intravascular coagulation, shock and death) leading to death when injected in most mammals [64]. Thanks to the development of more and more efficient systems today tests (LAL-test) for bacterial endotoxins (BET) can be completed before release of the batch of the ^{68}Ga-radiopharmaceuticals.

In contrary, the test for sterility of ^{68}Ga-radiopharmaceuticals via direct inoculation is necessarily retrospective nevertheless indispensable. Additionally, to the direct inoculation test the integrity of the sterile filter used for sterile filtration of the final product is performed. Due to the need for sterilization to obtain a sterile parenteral solution and the not applicability of autoclaving for short-living radiopharmaceuticals membrane filtration is normally the method of choice. The tests for the filter integrity (e.g. bubble point, diffusion rate, pressure hold) have the advantage that they can be completed before batch release.

10. *Radioactivity content/concentration*. Defines the activity, measured with a dose calibrator, within the volume of the final preparation.

11. *Specific radioactivity*. The specific radioactivity (activity of the radionuclide per unit mass either of the element or the desired chemical form) is calculated using the concentrations of radioactivity and the chemical form. Referring to the consensus nomenclature rules for radiopharmaceutical chemistry [65], the specific activity is expressed as measured activity per gram of compound (e.g. MBq/μg), while it is called molar activity when expressing the measured

activity per mole of compound (MBq/nmol) [65]. As gallium-68 requires a complex ligand which is normally not fully removed during the final product purification, the measured specific or molar activity is lower than actual. Then the correct terms are apparent specific or molar activity [65].

The specific or molar activity is always given with reference date and time.

8.1 Generator obtained gallium-68

For gallium-68 obtained from a $^{68}Ge/^{68}Ga$-generator, the Ph. Eur. contains a distinct monograph (#2464). This monograph specifies the quality characteristics of ^{68}Ga chloride solutions for radiolabeling independently if obtained directly from a generator or after post-processing the generator eluate. If a further purification of the generator eluate is performed, this has to be stated on the label.

Use of generator-produced gallium-68 in the USA is regulated under 10 CFR 35. 1000 and 10 CFR 30.33 [66] (**Table 3**).

For incoming starting materials, the GMP guidelines prescribe certain handling procedures to ensure their quality and suitability. For material acceptance of an incoming new $^{68}Ge/^{68}Ga$-generator, minimum controls are needed. This include the conformation of the radionuclide identity, ^{68}Ge-breakthrough and of activity stated in the Certificate of Analysis (CoA) all verified by activity measurement if possible [60]. Establishment of additional acceptance criteria may be required.

Nevertheless, the ^{68}Ga-eluate used for radiolabeling should meet those specifications (**Table 4**), their verification is in clinical routine not possible for every production. This results from the different production routes of ^{68}Ga-radiopharmaceuticals, which do not intend or allow an intervention for sampling of the eluate. Thus, the quality control of the starting material gallium-68 or of the final radiopharmaceuticals is allowed. This should include at least tests for ^{68}Ge-breakthrough, radionuclidic purity, radiochemical purity and chemical purity.

8.2 Cyclotron produced gallium-68

When produced via accelerator, the presence of the radioisotopes gallium-66 and gallium-67 is difficult to avoid due to zinc-66 and zinc-67 contaminating the

WHAT?	HOW?	LIMITS
Appearance	Visual inspection	Clear, colorless solution
pH	pH indicator strips	<2
Radionuclide identity	Half-life determination	62–74 min
	γ-spectrometry	511, (1022), 1077, (18,839 keV
Radionuclidic purity	γ-spectrometry	<0.1% long living impurities
		<0.001% germanium-68
Radiochemical purity	TLC	>95% $^{68}Ga(III)$
Chemical purity	ICP-AES/ICP-MS	<10 μg/GBq Fe
		<10 μg/GBq Zn
Bacterial Endotoxins	LAL test	≤175 EU/total volume

Table 3.
Quality control specifications for diluted hydrochloric solutions of generator produced gallium-68 as defined by the Ph. Eur. (monograph #2464) [59].

Manufacturer	Type	Maximum nominal activity
Eckert & Ziegler (Germany)	GalliaPharm®	2.4 GBq
	IGG100	2.4 GBq
Obninsk Cyclotron Ltd. (Russia)		3.7 GBq
IRE Elit (Belgium)	Galio Eo®	1.85 GBq
	Galli Ad®	1.85 GBq
ITG (Germany)		2 GBq
iThemba Labs (South Africa)		1.85 GBq
Pars Isotopes (Iran)	Pars-GalluGEN	2.59 GBq

Table 4.
In all conscience a list of ^{68}*Ge/*^{68}*Ga-generators available.*

target material. In return, germanium-68 is absent. Therefore, quality control and specifications for radionuclidic impurities are different to generator-produced gallium-68.

For gallium-68 obtained from a cyclotron, a new monograph (#3109) is already submitted for adoption to the Ph. Eur. [67]. This monograph specifies the quality characteristics of ^{68}Ga-chloride solutions for radiolabeling obtained by irradiation of enriched zinc-68 in an accelerator with subsequent isolation of gallium-68 in acidic solution (**Table 5**).

Similar to generator-produced gallium-68, quality control can be performed of the starting material obtained via cyclotron or on the final radiopharmaceutical. If quality control of the final radiopharmaceuticals performed, it should include at least tests for ^{68}Ge-breakthrough, radionuclidic purity, radiochemical purity and chemical purity.

8.3 ^{68}Ga-Radiopharmaceuticals

As an example for the specifications and limitations for a ^{68}Ga-radiopharmaceutical quality control as requested by the monograph #2464 of the

WHAT?	HOW?	LIMITS
Appearance	Visual inspection	Clear, colorless solution
pH	pH indicator strips	<2
Radionuclide identity	Half-life determination	62–74 min
	γ-spectrometry	511, (1022), 1077, (18,839 keV
Radionuclidic purity	γ-spectrometry	<0.1% long living impurities
		<2% gallium-66 & gallium-67
Radiochemical purity	TLC	>95% ^{68}Ga(III)
Chemical purity	ICP-AES/ICP-MS	<10 µg/GBq Fe
		<10 µg/GBq Zn
Bacterial Endotoxins	LAL test	≤175 EU/total volume

Table 5.
Quality control specifications for diluted hydrochloric solutions of accelerator-produced gallium-68 as defined by a draft of a monograph for the Ph. Eur. Submitted for adoption (#3109) [67].

WHAT?	HOW?	LIMITS
Appearance	Visual inspection	Clear, colorless solution
pH	pH indicator strips	< 2
Radionuclide identity	Half-life determination	62 to 74 min
	γ-spectrometry	511, (1022), 1077, (18,839 keV
Radionuclidic purity	γ-spectrometry	<0.1% long living impurities
		<0.001% germanium-68
Radiochemical purity	TLC	>91%
	TLC	<3% [^{68}Ga]Ga in colloidal form
	HPLC	<2% [^{68}Ga]Ga^{3+}
Chemical purity	ICP-AES/ICP-MS	<10 µg/GBq Fe
		<10 µg/GBq Zn
	HPLC	<50 µg/V DOTA-TOC and metal complexes of DOTA-TOC
	TLC	<200 µg/V HEPES
	GC	<10% V/V and <2.5 g per administration
Bacterial endotoxins	LAL test	≤175 EU/total volume
Sterility	Direct inoculation	sterile

Table 6.
Quality control specifications [^{68}Ga]Ga-DOTA-TOC as given by the Ph. Eur. For generator-produced gallium-68 (monograph #2464) [59].

Ph. Eur. [^{68}Ga]Ga-DOTA-TOC is provided [59]. It has to be noted, that monograph #2464 is currently under revision which can lead to different limits in feature (**Table 6**).

9. Regulatory aspects: the most important at the end

The quality control for a certain ^{68}Ga-radiopharmaceutical depends on the production route of gallium-68, the synthesis route of the radiopharmaceutical as well as of the relevant legislation.

As descripted in Section 7.2, the respective production route leads to different radionuclidic impurities (germanium-68 vs. gallium-66 & gallium-67) that need to take into account for the final product specifications. However, this is not yet implemented in the pharmacopeias but is in part already in progress. For example, the monograph for [^{68}Ga]Ga-DOTA-TOC (#2464) of the Ph. Eur. is currently in revision to take into account the cyclotron production of gallium-68 [68].

In general, the quality of the final radiopharmaceutical needs to fulfill all specifications given by the relevant legislation or pharmacopeia independent from the synthesis route. Nevertheless, it may be possible to dispense individual tests given, for example, for licensed kit preparations. For example, the Ph. Eur. states in its general notices "An article is not of Pharmacopoeia quality unless it complies with all the requirements stated in the monograph. This does not imply that performance of all the tests in a monograph is necessarily a prerequisite for a manufacturer in assessing compliance with the Pharmacopoeia before release of a product. The manufacturer may obtain assurance that a product is of Pharmacopoeia quality on the basis of its design, together with its control strategy and data derived, for example, from validation studies of the manufacturing process" [59]. Further details can be found in the general chapter on extemporaneous preparation of radiopharmaceuticals (5.19) and the general monograph radiopharmaceutical preparations (#0125) [59].

Nevertheless, the competent authorities may request further quality control testing. Therefore, it is strongly recommended, especially in case of doubt, to consult the competent authorities.

The implementation of a new radiopharmaceutical into the certain pharmacopeias is a protracted process. Therefore, several commonly used ^{68}Ga-radiopharmaceuticals are not yet represented with own monographs in the pharmacopeias (e.g. [^{68}Ga]Ga-PSMA-11). Nevertheless, such radiopharmaceuticals can be produced with consideration of the general notices, texts, monographs and along the lines of, for example, the monograph for [^{68}Ga]Ga-DOTA-TOC. Again, in case of doubt, the competent authorities should be consulted.

10. Conclusion

Gallium-68 is a well-researched radionuclide with growing importance for clinical practice triggered by the development of new tracers expanding its application and the increasing demand for theranostic patient care.

Its availability via radionuclide generator in combination with comparably easy coordination chemistry enables a patient care even in places where the cyclotron-produced PET-radionuclides are unavailable and, in the case of NETs, enables patient care where no ^{18}F-alternative exists.

Acknowledgements

This work was supported by the Ministry of Science and Higher Education of the Russian Federation project RFMEFI60719X0301.

Conflict of interest

The authors declare no conflict of interest.

Abbreviations

AEX	anion-exchange
API	active pharmaceutical ingredient
BET	bacterial endotoxin test
CEX	cation-exchange
DMF	drug master file
EU	European Union
FDA	U.S. Food and Drug Administration
GC	gas chromatography
GMP	good manufacturing practice
HCl	hydrochloric acid
HPLC	high pressure liquid chromatography
ICP-AES	inductively coupled plasma atomic emission spectroscopy
ICP-MS	inductively coupled plasma mass spectrometry
ITG	Isotopen Technologien Garching

LAL-test	limulus amebocyte lysate test
M	molarity (mol/liter)
MA	marketing authorization
mCRPC	metastatic castrate-resistant prostate cancer
NET	neuroendocrine tumor
PC	prostate cancer
PET	positron emission tomography
Ph. Eur.	European pharmacopeia
pmol	picomol (10^{-12} mol).
QC	quality control
PRRT	peptide receptor radionuclide therapy
SPE	solid phase extraction
$T_{1/2}$	half-life
TLC	thin layer chromatography
USA	United States of America
U.S.	United States
USP	United States Pharmacopeia

Author details

Michael Meisenheimer[1*], Yury Saenko[2] and Elisabeth Eppard[3*]

1 Department of Nuclear Medicine, University Hospital Bonn, Germany

2 S.P. Kapitsa Research Institute of Technology, Ulyanovsk State University, Ulyanovsk, Russia

3 Positronpharma SA, Providencia, Chile

*Address all correspondence to: michael.meisenheimer@ukbonn.de and eeppard@positronpharma.cl

IntechOpen

© 2019 The Author(s). Licensee IntechOpen. This chapter is distributed under the terms of the Creative Commons Attribution License (http://creativecommons.org/licenses/by/3.0), which permits unrestricted use, distribution, and reproduction in any medium, provided the original work is properly cited.

References

[1] Werner RA, Bluemel C, Allen-Auerbach MS, Higuchi T, Herrmann K. ^{68}Gallium- and ^{90}Yttrium−/ ^{177}Lutetium: "Theranostic twins" for diagnosis and treatment of NETs. Annals of Nuclear Medicine. 2015;**29**(1):1-7

[2] Strosberg J, Wolin E, Chasen B, Kulke M, Bushnell D, Caplin M, et al. Health-related quality of life in patients with progressive Midgut neuroendocrine tumors treated with 177Lu-Dotatate in the phase III NETTER-1 trial. Journal of Clinical Oncology. 2018;**36**(25):2578-2584

[3] Strosberg J, El-Haddad G, Wolin E, Hendifar A, Yao J, Chasen B, et al. Phase 3 trial of 177Lu-Dotatate for Midgut neuroendocrine tumors. The New England Journal of Medicine. 2017;**376**(2):125-135

[4] Paganelli G, Sansovini M, Ambrosetti A, Severi S, Monti M, Scarpi E, et al. 177 Lu-Dota-octreotate radionuclide therapy of advanced gastrointestinal neuroendocrine tumors: Results from a phase II study. European Journal of Nuclear Medicine and Molecular Imaging. 2014;**41**(10):1845-1851

[5] Mahajan S, O'Donoghue J, Weber W, Bodei L. Integrating early rapid post-peptide receptor radionuclide therapy quality assurance scan into the outpatient setting. Journal of Nuclear Medicine and Radiation Therapy. 2019;**10**(1):395

[6] Carlsen EA, Fazio N, Granberg D, Grozinsky-Glasberg S, Ahmadzadehfar H, Grana CM, et al. Peptide receptor radionuclide therapy in gastroenteropancreatic NEN G3: A multicenter cohort study. Endocrine-Related Cancer. 2019;**26**(2):227-239

[7] Capdevila J, Fazio N, Lopez C, Teule A, Valle JW, Tafuto S, et al. 1307OEfficacy of lenvatinib in patients with advanced pancreatic (panNETs) and gastrointestinal (giNETs) grade 1/2 (G1/G2) neuroendocrine tumors: Results of the international phase II TALENT trial (GETNE 1509). Annals of Oncology. 2018;**29**(suppl_8)

[8] Bodei L, Cremonesi M, Grana CM, Fazio N, Iodice S, Baio SM, et al. Peptide receptor radionuclide therapy with ^{177}Lu-DOTATATE: The IEO phase I-II study. European Journal of Nuclear Medicine and Molecular Imaging. 2011;**38**(12):2125-2135

[9] Sorbye H, Welin S, Langer SW, Vestermark LW, Holt N, Osterlund P, et al. Predictive and prognostic factors for treatment and survival in 305 patients with advanced gastrointestinal neuroendocrine carcinoma (WHO G3): The NORDIC NEC study. Annals of Oncology. 2013;**24**(1):152-160

[10] Gleason GI. A positron cow. The International Journal of Applied Radiation and Isotopes. 1960;**8**(2-3):90-94

[11] Breeman WAP, Jong M, Blois E, Bernard BF, Konijnenberg M, Krenning EP. Radiolabelling DOTA-peptides with ^{68}Ga. European Journal of Nuclear Medicine and Molecular Imaging. 2005;**32**(4):478-485

[12] Velikyan I, Beyer GJ, Langström B. Microwave-supported preparation of ^{68}Ga bioconjugates with high specific radioactivity. Bioconjugate Chemistry. 2004;**15**(3):554-560

[13] Meyer G-J, Mäcke H, Schuhmacher J, Knapp WH, Hofmann M. ^{68}Ga-labelled DOTA-derivatised peptide ligands. European Journal of Nuclear Medicine and Molecular Imaging. 2004;**31**(8):1097-1104

[14] Lenzo NP, Meyrick D, Turner JH. Review of Gallium-68 PSMA PET/CT

imaging in the management of prostate cancer. Diagnostics (Basel). 2018;**8**(1):16

[15] Raj N, Reidy-Lagunes D. The role of 68Ga-DOTATATE positron emission tomography/computed tomography in well-differentiated neuroendocrine tumors: A case-based approach illustrates potential benefits and challenges. Pancreas. 2018;**47**(1):1-5

[16] Jansen TJP, van Lith SAM, Boss M, Brom M, Joosten L, Béhé M, et al. Exendin-4 analogs in insulinoma theranostics. Journal of Labelled Compounds and Radiopharmaceuticals. 2019;**62**(10):656-672

[17] Zhang J, Mao F, Niu G, Peng L, Lang L, Li F, et al. 68Ga-BBN-RGD PET/CT for GRPR and integrin αvβ3 imaging in patients with breast cancer. Theranostics. 2018;**8**(4):1121-1130

[18] Zhang J, Li D, Lang L, Zhu Z, Wang L, Wu P, et al. 68Ga-NOTA-Aca-BBN(7-14) PET/CT in healthy volunteers and glioma patients. Journal of Nuclear Medicine. 2016;**57**(1):9-14

[19] Velikyan I, Schweighöfer P, Feldwisch J, Seemann J, Frejd FY, Lindman H, et al. Diagnostic HER2-binding radiopharmaceutical, 68GaGa-ABY-025, for routine clinical use in breast cancer patients. American Journal of Nuclear Medicine and Molecular Imaging. 2019;**9**(1):12-23

[20] Schoffelen R, Sharkey RM, Goldenberg DM, Franssen G, McBride WJ, Rossi EA, et al. Pretargeted immuno-positron emission tomography imaging of carcinoembryonic antigen-expressing tumors with a bispecific antibody and a 68Ga- and 18F-labeled hapten peptide in mice with human tumor xenografts. Molecular Cancer Therapeutics. 2010;**9**(4):1019-1027

[21] IAEA. Gallium-68 Cyclotron Production. Vienna: International Atomic Energy Agency; 2019

[22] Velikyan I. Positron emitting 68GaGa-based imaging agents: Chemistry and diversity. Medicinal Chemistry. 2011;**7**(5):345-379

[23] McCutchan EA. Nuclear data sheets for a = 68. Nuclear Data Sheets. 2012;**113**(6-7):1735-1870

[24] Available from: http://www.nndc.bnl.gov/chart

[25] Razbash AA, Sevastianov YG, Krasnov NN, Leonov AI, Pavlekin VE, editor. Germanium-68 row of products. In: Proceedings of the 5th International Conference on Isotopes, 5ICI; Brussels, Belgium; 2005

[26] Dash A, Chakravarty R. Radionuclide generators: The prospect of availing PET radiotracers to meet current clinical needs and future research demands. American Journal of Nuclear Medicine and Molecular Imaging. 2019;**9**(1):30-66

[27] Mueller D, Klette I, Baum RP, Gottschaldt M, Schultz MK, Breeman WAP. Simplified NaCl based ^{68}Ga concentration and labeling procedure for rapid synthesis of ^{68}Ga radiopharmaceuticals in high radiochemical purity. Bioconjugate Chemistry. 2012;**23**(8):1712-1717

[28] Eppard E, Wuttke M, Nicodemus PL, Rösch F. Ethanol-based post-processing of generator derived ^{68}Ga towards kit-type preparation of ^{68}Ga-radiopharmaceuticals. Journal of Nuclear Medicine. 2014;**55**:1023-1028

[29] Zhernosekov KP, Filosofov DV, Baum RP, Aschoff P, Bihl H, Razbash AA, et al. Processing of generator-produced ^{68}Ga for medical application. Journal of Nuclear Medicine. 2007;**48**(10):1741-1748

[30] Mueller D, Klette I, Baum RP. The combined cationic-anionic purification of the ^{68}Ge/^{68}Ga generator eluate

for the labelling of fragile peptides. World Journal of Nuclear Medicine. 2011;**10**(1):73-89

[31] Loktionova NS, Belozub AN, Filosofov DV, Zhernosekov KP, Wagner T, Türler A, et al. Improved column-based radiochemical processing of the generator produced ^{68}Ga. Applied Radiation and Isotopes. 2011;**69**(7):942-946

[32] Gilly LJ, Henriet GA, Alves MP, Capron PC. Absolute cross sections and excitation functions for (d, p) and (d, 2n) reactions on Mn55 , Cu63, Cu65 , Zn66 , and Zn68 between 3 and 11.6 MeV. Physics Review. 1963;**131**(4):1727-1731

[33] Szelecsényi F, Kovács Z, Nagatsu K, Fukumura K, Suzuki K, Mukai K. Investigation of direct production of 68 Ga with low energy multiparticle accelerator. Radiochimica Acta. 2012;**100**(1):5-11

[34] Ugur Ö, Kothari PJ, Finn RD, Zanzonico P, Ruan S, Guenther I, et al. Ga-66 labeled somatostatin analogue DOTA-DPhe 1 -Tyr 3 -octreotide as a potential agent for positron emission tomography imaging and receptor mediated internal radiotherapy of somatostatin receptor positive tumors. Nuclear Medicine and Biology. 2002;**29**(2):147-157

[35] Lewis MR, Reichert DE, Laforest R, Margenau WH, Shefer RE, Klinkowstein RE, et al. Production and purification of gallium-66 for preparation of tumor-targeting radiopharmaceuticals. Nuclear Medicine and Biology. 2002;**29**(6):701-706

[36] Sadeghi M, Mokhtari L. Rapid separation of 67,68Ga from 68Zn target using precipitation technique. Journal of Radioanalytical and Nuclear Chemistry. 2010;**284**(2):471-473

[37] Alves F, Alves VHP, Do Carmo SJC, Neves ACB, Silva M, Abrunhosa AJ. Production of copper-64 and gallium-68 with a medical cyclotron using liquid targets. Modern Physics Letters A. 2017;**32**(17):1740013

[38] Lin M, Waligorski GJ, Lepera CG. Production of curie quantities of 68Ga with a medical cyclotron via the 68Zn(p,n)68Ga reaction. Applied Radiation and Isotopes. 2018;**133**:1-3

[39] Nair M. Cyclotron production and automated new 2-column processing of [68Ga]$GaCl_3$. European Journal of Nuclear Medicine and Molecular Imaging. 2017;**44**(Suppl 2):119-956

[40] Oehlke E, Hoehr C, Hou X, Hanemaayer V, Zeisler S, Adam MJ, et al. Production of Y-86 and other radiometals for research purposes using a solution target system. Nuclear Medicine and Biology. 2015;**42**(11):842-849

[41] Pandey MK, Bansal A, Engelbrecht HP, Byrne JF, Packard AB, DeGrado TR. Improved production and processing of ^{89}Zr using a solution target. Nuclear Medicine and Biology. 2016;**43**(1):97-100

[42] Pandey MK, Byrne JF, Jiang H, Packard AB, DeGrado TR. Cyclotron production of (68)Ga via the (68) Zn(p,n)(68)Ga reaction in aqueous solution. American Journal of Nuclear Medicine and Molecular Imaging. 2014;**4**(4):303-310

[43] Pandey MK, Byrne JF, Schlasner KN, Schmit NR, DeGrado TR. Cyclotron production of ^{68}Ga in a liquid target: Effects of solution composition and irradiation parameters. Nuclear Medicine and Biology. 2019;(**74-75**):49-55

[44] Engle JW, Lopez-Rodriguez V, Gaspar-Carcamo RE, Valdovinos HF, Valle-Gonzalez M, Trejo-Ballado F, et al. Very high specific activity $^{66/68}$Ga from zinc targets for PET. Applied Radiation and Isotopes. 2012;**70**(8):1792-1796

[45] Breeman WAP, de Blois E, Sze Chan H, Konijnenberg M, Kwekkeboom DJ, Krenning EP. ^{68}Ga-labeled DOTA-peptides and ^{68}Ga-labeled radiopharmaceuticals for positron emission tomography: Current status of research, clinical applications, and future perspectives. Seminars in Nuclear Medicine. 2011;**41**(4):314-321

[46] Eder M, Wängler B, Knackmuss S, LeGall F, Little M, Haberkorn U, et al. Tetrafluorophenolate of HBED-CC: A versatile conjugation agent for ^{68}Ga-labeled small recombinant antibodies. European Journal of Nuclear Medicine and Molecular Imaging. 2008;**35**(10):1878-1886

[47] Mathias CJ, Green MA. A convenient route to [68Ga]Ga-MAA for use as a particulate PET perfusion tracer. Applied Radiation and Isotopes. 2008;**66**(12):1910-1912

[48] Riss PJ, Kroll C, Nagel V, Rösch F. NODAPA-OH and NODAPA-(NCS)n: Synthesis, 68Ga-radiolabelling and in vitro characterisation of novel versatile bifunctional chelators for molecular imaging. Bioorganic and Medicinal Chemistry Letters. 2008;**18**(20):5364-5367

[49] Rösch F, Riss PJ. The renaissance of the ^{68}Ge/^{68}Ga radionuclide generator initiates new developments in ^{68}Ga radiopharmaceutical chemistry. Current Topics in Medicinal Chemistry. 2010;**10**(16):1633-1668

[50] Šimeček J, Hermann P, Wester H-J, Notni J. How is (68)Ga labeling of macrocyclic chelators influenced by metal ion contaminants in (68)Ge/(68) Ga generator eluates? ChemMedChem. 2013;**8**(1):95-103

[51] Velikyan I, Lendvai G, Välilä M, Roivainen A, Yngve U, Bergström M, et al. Microwave accelerated ^{68}Ga-labelling of oligonucleotides. Journal of Labelled Compounds and Radiopharmaceuticals. 2004;**47**(1):79-89

[52] Sun Y, Anderson CJ, Pajeau TS, Reichert DE, Hancock RD, Motekaitis RJ, et al. Indium (III) and gallium (III) complexes of bis(aminoethanethiol) ligands with different denticities: Stabilities, molecular modeling, and in vivo behavior. Journal of Medicinal Chemistry. 1996;**39**(2):458-470

[53] Wadas TJ, Wong EH, Weisman GR, Anderson CJ. Coordinating radiometals of copper, gallium, indium, yttrium, and zirconium for PET and SPECT imaging of disease. Chemical Reviews. 2010;**110**(5):2858-2902

[54] Taliaferro CH, Martell AE. New multidentate ligands. Xxvi. N,N' -BIS(2-hydroxybenzyl)ethylenediamine- N,N' -bis(methylenephosphonic acid monomethyl ester), and N,N' -bis(2-hydroxybenzyl) ethylenediamine- N,N' -bis (methylenephosphonic acid monoethyl ester): New chelating ligands for trivalent metal ions. Journal of Coordination Chemistry. 1984;**13**(3):249-264

[55] https://www.gmp-compliance.org/guidelines/gmp-guidelines

[56] Martin R, Jüttler S, Müller M, Wester H-J. Cationic eluate pretreatment for automated synthesis of [^{68}Ga] CPCR4.2. Nuclear Medicine and Biology. 2014;**41**(1):84-89

[57] Aslani A, Snowdon GM, Bailey DL, Schembri GP, Bailey EA, Roach PJ. Gallium-68 DOTATATE production with automated PET radiopharmaceutical synthesis system: A three year experience. Asia Oceania Journal of Nuclear Medicine and Biology. 2014;**2**(2):75-86

[58] Iori M, Capponi PC, Rubagotti S, Esposizione LR, Seemann J, Pitzschler R, et al. Labelling of 90 Y- and 177 Lu-DOTA-bioconjugates for targeted radionuclide therapy: A comparison among manual,

semiautomated, and fully automated synthesis. Contrast Media and Molecular Imaging. 2017;(7):1-12

[59] European Pharmacopoeia, 10th Edition 2019. Subscription to Main Volume + Supplement 1 + Supplement 2. 1st ed. Stuttgart: Deutscher Apotheker Verlag; 2019

[60] IAEA. Quality Control in the Production of Radiopharmaceuticals. Vienna: International Atomic Energy Agency; 2018

[61] WHO Pharmacopoeia Library. Available from: http://apps.who.int/phint/en/p/docf/

[62] Langille SE. Particulate matter in injectable drug products. PDA Journal of Pharmaceutical Science and Technology. 2013;**67**(3):186-200

[63] Pauli GF, Chen S-N, Simmler C, Lankin DC, Gödecke T, Jaki BU, et al. Importance of purity evaluation and the potential of quantitative ^{1}H NMR as a purity assay. Journal of Medicinal Chemistry. 2014;**57**(22):9220-9231

[64] Todar K, Madison WI. Bacterial Endotoxin. Available from: http://textbookofbacteriology.net/endotoxin.html

[65] Coenen HH, Gee AD, Adam M, Antoni G, Cutler CS, Fujibayashi Y, et al. Consensus nomenclature rules for radiopharmaceutical chemistry - setting the record straight. Nuclear Medicine and Biology. 2017;**55**:v-xi

[66] U.S. Nuclear regulatory Commision. Germanium-68/Gallium-68 Pharmaceutical Grade Generators Licensing Guidance. 2019. Available from: www.nrc.gov/docs/ML1910/ML19106A367.pdf

[67] Council of Europe. Pharmeuropa Online 30.4. Available from: http://pharmeuropa.edqm.eu/home/

[68] EDQM. Knowledge Database. Available from: https://extranet.edqm.eu/4DLink1/4DCGI/Web_View/mono/2464

Chapter 3

Parathyroid Scintigraphy

Albena Dimitrova Botushanova and Nikolay Petrov Botushanov

Abstract

The visualization of abnormal parathyroid glands is difficult due to their variations in number and localization. Noninvasive parathyroid imaging studies include ^{99m}Tc-sestamibi scintigraphy, ultrasonography, computed tomography scanning, magnetic resonance imaging, and positron emission tomography. There is a general consensus that the most sensitive and specific imaging modality, especially when it is combined with single-photon emission CT is the scintigraphy with ^{99m}Tc-sestamibi or ^{99m}Tc-tetrofosmin. ^{99m}Tc-sestamibi scintigraphy significantly increases the role of preoperative scintigraphy in patients with hyperparathyroidism and allows unilateral surgical approach with minimally invasive parathyroidectomy to be used. Generally, three protocols with the use of two radiopharmaceuticals, ^{99m}Tc-sestamibi or ^{99m}Tc-tetrofosmin, are most widely applied: single-phase dual-isotope subtraction, dual-phase single-isotope and combination of both. Each one of them has specific advantages and disadvantages. While single parathyroid adenomas are localized with greater precision, hyperfunctioning parathyroid hyperplastic cells represent a real challenge to the imaging modalities. Several factors can influence the radionuclide uptake in pathologically changed parathyroid cells, like the size, the level of their functional activity, the quantity of oxyphilic cells, mitochondria, P glycoprotein and other MDR gene products.

Keywords: parthyroid scintigraphy, SPECT, ^{99m}Tc-sestamibi, ^{99m}Tc-tetrofosmin, ^{99m}Tc pertechnetate

1. Introduction

Noninvasive parathyroid imaging studies include technetium (^{99m}Tc) sestamibi scintigraphy, ultrasonography (US), computed tomography (CT) scanning, magnetic resonance imaging (MRI) and positron emission tomography (PET). Parathyroid glands need to be examined in case of a diagnosed hyperparathyroidism as a part of preoperative localization of the abnormal glands. Hyperparathyroidism is characterized by elevated parathyroid hormone (PTH) levels in the blood. Due to the underlying cause, it can be divided into primary and secondary. The primary hyperparathyroidism (PHPT) is due to excessive production of PTH from one or more abnormal parathyroid glands. Secondary hyperparathyroidism (SHPT) is a result of hypocalcemia caused by other concomitant diseases (end stage kidney renal disease, etc.). In SHPT usually more than one parathyroid glands are affected. Considered rare disease in the past, the incidence of PHPT has changed dramatically during the last 30 years with the introduction of routine calcium measurements in clinical practice, and is now considered to be approximately 42 per 100,000 persons. Women are affected more frequently than

IntechOpen

men, in a ratio of approximately 3:1. PHPT occurs predominantly in individuals in their middle years with a peak incidence between ages 50 and 60 years and can reach 4 cases per 1000 persons in women after their 60s. At the time of diagnosis, most patients with PHPT do not have classic symptoms like osteitis fibrosa cystica, nephrocalcinosis, nephrolithiasis or other signs associated with the disease. Symptomatic PHPT is now exception rather than the rule, with more than three-fourths of patients having no symptoms making detected changes of the blood values of calcium, phosphorus and parathyroid hormone (PTH) to be the only reason for diagnosis [1, 2]. By far, the most common lesion found in patients with PHPT is the solitary parathyroid adenoma, occurring in 85–90% of patients, while in the rest 10–15% primary hyperplasia of the parathyroid glands is present [3]. In the past the standard surgical approach for PHPT was the bilateral four-gland parathyroid exploration with the removal of each gland which showed changes macroscopically. While in most of the patients with PHPT only one parathyroid gland is being affected, the above mentioned surgical approach is inappropriate in all cases. Unilateral approaches are appealing in a disease in which only a single gland is involved. So nowadays, the currently most widely used surgical approach is the minimally invasive parathyroidectomy which is connected with less post-surgical complications and shortens the time of operation [4]. To be successful this procedure needs to rely on a precise preoperative localization of the abnormal parathyroid glands. That is, why preoperative parathyroid imaging gained so large importance. The rationale for locating abnormal parathyroid glands prior to surgery is that they can be notoriously unpredictable in their location.

2. Anatomy of the parathyroid glands

Parathyroid glands differ in shape and size. Typically four glands are present and are located adjacent to the dorsal surface of the thyroid lobes-two upper and two lower pairs. Normal glands tend to be flat and oval and normal measurements are 3 × 5 × 7 mm [5]. The combined weight of all parathyroid glans is 90–130 mg and the superior glands are smaller than the inferior [6, 7]. Autopsy series demonstrate that four glands are found in 91% in subjects, five glands in 4%, and three glands in 5% [8]. Approximately 5% of humans have supernumerary (more than four) parathyroid glands [9]. Supernumerary glands are most commonly found within the thymus. Although gland distribution may deviate widely, the superior parathyroid glands, originating from the fourth pharyngeal pouch, are commonly found along the posterior surface of the upper two-thirds of the thyroid gland (92%). The inferior parathyroid glands have a more variable distribution than the superior ones. They originate from the third pharyngeal pouch together with the thymus. They migrate caudally until they reach the lower pole of the thyroid gland and 17% of them touch the inferior border of the thyroid gland, 26% are within the superior horn of the thymus, and 2% are in the mediastinal thymus [10]. The variable anatomic distribution makes the inferior glands more difficult to locate than the superior ones. Histologically parathyroid glands are made of chief, oxyphillic and transient oxyphillic cells mixed with fat tissue. Chief cells produce PTH. The oxyphillic cells which are rich of mitochondria are with poorly defined function [11].

3. Noninvasive parathyroid imaging

The normal parathyroid glands cannot be visualized. The lack of the perfect imaging method for precise localization of parathyroid adenomas had led to search for an alternative imaging techniques. Ultrasonography (US) is one of the most widely used procedures. Because of the great anatomic variations of the parathyroid glands, their small sizes, the presence of more than one abnormal gland and the higher frequency of concomitant morphological changes of the thyroid gland, US proved to be specific but with low sensitivity. The success of US is highly operator dependent [12]. Rapid spiral thin-slice CT scanning of the neck and mediastinum with evaluation of axial, coronal and sagittal views can add much to the search for elusive parathyroid tissue [13]. MRI can also identify abnormal parathyroid tissue, but it is time consuming and expensive. It is also less sensitive than other modalities. It can nonetheless be useful when the search with the other noninvasive approaches has been unsuccessful. PET/CT can be used, but like MRI, it is expensive and does not have the kind of experiential basis that make it attractive. There are limiting data for using PET/CT in parathyroid imaging. PET with ^{18}F-fluorodeoxyglucose (^{18}F-FDG) was used with varying success. One study showed that ^{18}F-FDG PET was more sensitive but less specific than ^{99m}Tc-sestamibi SPECT [14]. Others reported very low sensitivity for detecting abnormal parathyroid glands [15]. Using PET with ^{11}C-methionine in parathyroid examination has been studied in some patients but because of the very short half-life of ^{11}C-methionine, only 20 min its use is limited only to nuclear medicine centers located near to a cyclotron. There is a general consensus that the most sensitive and specific imaging modality, especially when it is combined with single-photon emission CT (SPECT) is the scintigraphy with ^{99m}Tc-sestamibi or ^{99m}Tc-tetrofosmin.

4. Parathyrod scintigraphy

Historically, the success of scintigraphy had been compromised by the failure of finding a pharmaceutical agent with specific topic accumulation in parathyroid glands and their close proximity to the thyroid gland. That is why to find a reliable method to differentiate both glands on scintigraphy was crucial. This was first achieved by a combined use of two radionuclides with different uptake in the thyroid and parathyroid cells. The latter allowed to perform a subtraction of the obtained images of both glands and to visualize only the abnormal parathyroid gland, but this proved to be time consuming and with greate radiation exposure to the patients. The first widely used radionuclide for detecting hyperfunctioning parathyroid glands during the 80s was ^{201}Thallium chloride (^{201}Tl). ^{201}Tl chloride accumulates equally in thyroid and parathyroid cells. To make differentiation possible, its application was followed by an injection of ^{99m}Tc pertechnetate, with predominant thyroid uptake. Then ^{99m}Tc pertechnetate thyroid images were digitally subtracted from the images obtained with ^{201}Tl chloride to allow visualization only of the parathyroid glands [16].

Introduced in clinical practice by Coakley et al. [17], the ^{99m}Tc-sestamibi scintigraphy significantly increased the role of preoperative scintigraphy in patients with hyperparathyroidism. Firstly used as a cardiotropic agent this radionuclide showed increased accumulation in a variety of benign and malignant tumors. ^{99m}Tc-sestamibi consists of lipophilic cationic molecules. After being intravenously injected these molecules distribute throughout the body accordingly to the local blood supply and by passive diffusion through cell's membrane accumulate intracellularly into the mitochondria [18, 19]. Normally ^{99m}Tc-sestamibi distributes in parotid and submandibular salivary glands, thyroid gland, the heart and the liver, but not in normal parathyroid glands. Visualization of parathyroid adenomas and hyperplastic parathyroid glands depends on the presence of oxyphillic cells, which are rich of mitochondria. The cells of parathyroid adenomas have plenty of mitochondria [20], while the normal parathyroid cells do not [21]. The highest rates of uptake of ^{99m}Tc-sestamibi are seen in the solitary adenomas of the parathyroid glands [22]. Not only the amount of intracellular mitochondria is important but also the quantity of oxyphillic cells in the tumors. If the percentage of oxyphillic cells exceeded 25%, accumulation of ^{99m}Tc-sestamibi was observed in 78% of parathyroid adenomas. Also false negative results are possible if the oxyphillic cells do not content sufficient amount of mitochondria [23]. Accumulation of ^{99m}Tc-sestamibi into the cells also can be influenced by their metabolic activity, the weight and the size of the tumor. This new radionuclide rapidly replaced ^{201}Tl chloride because it showed better quality of the images and higher sensitivity for detecting abnormal parathyroid glands, with less radiation exposure [24].

^{99m}Tc-tetrofosmin another myocardial perfusion agent was also used for visualizing parathyroid glands in scintigraphy, but the data for its use so far are limited. ^{99m}Tc-tetrofosmin shows some similarities with ^{99m}Tc-sestamibi although the way of accumulation is different and it is retained mainly in the cytosol rather than in the mitochondria of the target cells. When used for parathyroid scintigraphy ^{99m}Tc-tetrofosmin shows slower washout from the thyroid gland, which makes it unsuitable for single-isotope dual-phase scintigraphy [25]. Nevertheless its sensitivity increases when used in combination with SPECT. Several studies [26, 27] of the diagnostic value of ^{99m}Tc-tetrofosmin scintigraphy for topic localization of the hyperfunctioning parathyroid glands in patients with PHPT, showed that this method was useful for the clinical practice and that the accumulation of ^{99m}Tc-tetrofosmin depends on the weight of the tumor and the level of PTH.

4.1 Protocols for nuclear medicine examination of parathyroid glands

Generally three protocols are most widely used: single-phase dual-isotope subtraction, dual-phase single-isotope and combination of both [28].

In single-phase dual-isotope modality two types of radiopharmaceuticals with different organ uptake are used. One isotope (^{99m}Tc-sestamibi or ^{99m}Tc-tetrofosmin) with equal thyroid and parathyroid glands accumulation and another (^{123}I or ^{99m}Tc-pertechnetate) with predominant uptake in the thyroid gland are applied consecutively. The obtained images are digitally subtracted and if there is a residual radionuclide accumulation on the subtracted images a hyperfunctioning parathyroid gland can be suspected [28]. Disadvantages of this method are the use of two radionuclides, the necessity of full collaboration from the patient's side to stay calm and motionless during the examination and the need of very precise positioning of the patient. In addition there is an increase possibility for the presence of artifacts on the subtracted images [29, 30].

The rationale of the single-isotope protocol is based upon the different washout periods of the radionuclide from the thyroid and parathyroid glands. In this method, after an injection of a single radionuclide, early (at 10–15 min) and late (at 1.5–3 h) images are obtained [28].

There are a very few studies directly comparing the results from single-isotope dual-phase modality with single-phase dual-isotope subtractional scintigraphy and the results are inconclusive [31, 32]. So far there is no clear confirmed advantages of one type over another.

4.1.1 Preparation of the patient

No preliminary preparation of the patients before performing single isotope dual-phase scintigraphy is necessary. In subtractional modality some preliminary conditions should be followed such as: discontinuation of Levothyroxine or Iodine containing drugs minimum 20 days before the examination. A case history of every patient about the duration of the disease, any concomitant diseases and medications, especially drugs that could possibly interfere with the calcium-phosphate homeostasis, and family history should be taken.

4.1.2 Radiopharmaceuticals

^{99m}Tc-sestamibi and ^{99m}Tc-tetrofosmin: they are applied intravenously from 740 to 1110 MBq (20–30 mCi).

^{99m}Tc-pertechnetate has a half-life of 6 h and possesses energy of 140 keV. It is used for visualization of the thyroid gland because it accumulates in a functioning thyroid cells. Intravenously ^{99m}Tc-pertechnetate is applied form 74–350 MBq (2–10 mCi).

4.2 Single-isotope dual-phase scintigraphy with ^{99m}Tc-sestamibi and ^{99m}Tc-tetrofosmin

4.2.1 Single-isotope dual-phase scintigraphy with ^{99m}Tc-sestamibi

^{99m}Tc-sestamibi accumulates in the thyroid and parathyroid glands, but the washout time from both glands differs, showing faster disappearing from the thyroid and retention in parathyroid cells. This allows successful visualization of pathologically changed parathyroid glands on the obtained later images—1.5–2 h after the injection of the radionuclide. This different retention time in both glands may be related to some down-regulation of the P-glycoprotein system in parathyroid adenomas, which delays washout of the nuclide [33]. Just the opposite, in parathyroid hyperplasia these so-called multidrug-related resistance molecules can be upregulated and can cause faster washout of ^{99m}Tc-sestamibi and lead to false negative results [34, 35].

To avoid this disadvantage and to improve sensitivity and specificity, the use of single-isotope dual phase (early and late) scintigraphy, based upon the suggestion that ^{99m}Tc-sestamibi is washed out faster from the thyroid gland than from the hyperfunctioning parathyroid cells, is recommended [36]. This single-isotope dual phase scintigraphy gained popularity due to its convenience. The fact that ^{99m}Tc-sestamibi can also be accumulated in solitary thyroid nodules diminishes the specificity of this procedure, especially in areas with higher incidence of nodular goiter [37, 38]. Some parathyroid adenomas also show rapid washout of ^{99m}Tc-sestamibi and make their visualization difficult by this procedure [39]. This led to an introduction of a modified protocol for subtractional scintigraphy by adding a second radionuclide with a preferential accumulation in the thyroid tissue.

^{99m}Tc-sestamibi scintigraphy is generally regarded to be the most sensitive and specific imaging modality especially when it is combined with other imaging procedures. The combination of US examination with dual-isotope ^{99m}Tc pertechnetate/^{99m}Tc-sestamibi scintigraphy for preoperative localization of parathyroid adenomas leads to visualizing of the parathyroid adenomas in 95.2% of the cases (20 patients out of 21). Reaching such high diagnostic precision allows to minimize the extent of the surgical procedure and gives way to apply routinely and successfully minimally invasive parathyroidectomy only of the pathologically changed glands [40, 41].

Comparing different imaging methods, ^{99m}Tc-sestamibi scintigraphy has higher sensitivity and specificity than US and CT in discovering adenomas of the parathyroid glands. With regards to the hyperplasia of the parathyroid glands ^{99m}Tc-sestamibi scintigraphy shows to be of less value [42, 43]. Hyperplastic parathyroid glands are visualized in 10–62.5% of the cases [44, 45]. In multiple endocrine neoplasia syndrome (MEN), where hyperplasia of the parathyroid glands is common, only 55% of the abnormal glands are seen on ^{99m}Tc-sestamibi scintigraphy [42, 46, 47]. ^{99m}Tc-sestamibi scintigraphy shows to be highly effective in discovering ectopic hyperfunctioning parathyroid glands, which in some studies, are observed in approximately 20% of the cases with PHPT and represent a diagnostic and therapeutic challenge [48]. Visualizing small parathyroid adenomas represents a specific problem. One study showed, that in surgically removed adenomas weighted less than 0.5 g, preoperative US was negative, but ^{99m}Tc-sestamibi scintigraphy discovered adenomas in 87% of cases and the combination with SPECT increased sensitivity to 95% [21].

In patients with SHPT, seems to have a direct correlation between ^{99m}Tc-sestamibi uptake with the blood level of parathyroid hormone and the phase of the cells' cycles [49]. The lowest level of accumulation corresponds to G(0) phase and the highest to phase G(2) + S. No such correlation with the weight of the glands is found [49]. The fixation of the radionuclide depends on the functional status of the tissues, i.e., increased accumulation accompanies the cells' active growing phase or is directly connected to the state of autonomy of the parathyroid cells [46].

The reason why not all pathologically changed parathyroid glands accumulate radionuclide remains unclear. This may be due to the different degree of activity and proliferation of the cells of the parathyroid adenomas. It was suggested that there is a relationship between nuclide accumulation and the degree of autonomy of the cells of the adenoma, i.e., the loss of the suppressive effect of calcium upon the secretion of the parathyroid hormone. The cells of the parathyroid adenomas and these of the hyperplastic glands show higher threshold for calcium suppression or have no threshold at all in comparison with the normal parathyroid cells. Due to this fact, these cells secrete more PTH for any given blood calcium level, show higher metabolic rate and capability to accumulate more ^{99m}Tc-sestamibi. Hyperplastic parathyroid glands are to some extent with preserved functional regulation, respond to the normal suppressive stimuluses, have lower metabolic rate and accumulate less of the radionuclide.

Due to its higher affinity to the parathyroid adenomas, ^{99m}Tc-sestamibi scintigraphy was used in cases of relapse of the hyperparathyroidism after parathyroidectomy or after autotransplantation of parathyroid glands.

Nowadays, there are several imaging methods for discovering hyperplastic parathyroid glands. The results so far are inconclusive. The dual-phase ^{99m}Tc-sestamibi scintigraphy in preoperative localization of the hyperplastic parathyroid glands in patients with profound secondary hyperparathyroidism do not show high sensitivity, but is of help to discriminate between patients with nodular and diffuse hyperplasia [50].

The role of ^{99m}Tc-sestamibi scintigraphy in patients with end-stage renal disease and secondary hyperparathyroidism is still unclear. The uptake of ^{99m}Tc-sestamibi can be suppressed by the use of calcitriol in these patients. In one study [51] ^{99m}Tc-sestamibi scintigraphy managed to visualize 1 or more (maximum 3) parathyroid glands in most, but not in all patients on hemodialysis with PHT levels above 600 pg/ml. Performing suppressive test with calcitriol (2 mg of calcitriol applied i.v. after each hemodialysis for two consecutive weeks) showed suppression of ^{99m}Tc-sestamibi uptake at least in one parathyroid gland in 57% of the cases and full suppression in all glands in 36%. The basal level of PHT or its lowering after this test showed to be of no predictive value for the suppression of ^{99m}Tc-sestamibi uptake in the parathyroid glands. Because of its lower sensitivity, the ^{99m}Tc-sestamibi scintigraphy was found to be of limited value in preoperative evaluation in uremic patients with secondary hyperparathyroidism, but its significance grew up in localizing hyperfunctioning glands left after the first operation [51].

Single-isotope dual phase ^{99m}Tc-sestamibi scintigraphy is easily performed, and needs only application of ^{99m}Tc-sestamibi. After injection of the radiopharmaceutical, early (10–15 min), and late planar (1,5–3 h) images are obtained (**Figures 1** and **2**).

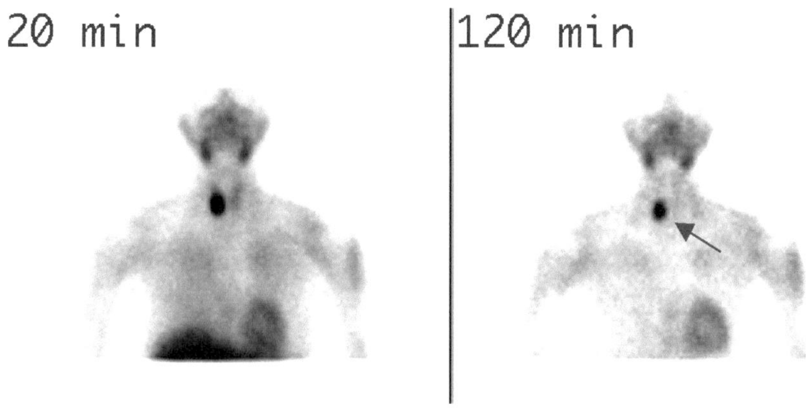

Figure 1.
Single-isotope dual-phase scintigraphy with ^{99m}Tc-sestamibi. The late image (120 min) shows a focus of a residual activity (arrow), caudally of the right thyroid lobe consistent with adenoma of the right lower parathyroid gland.

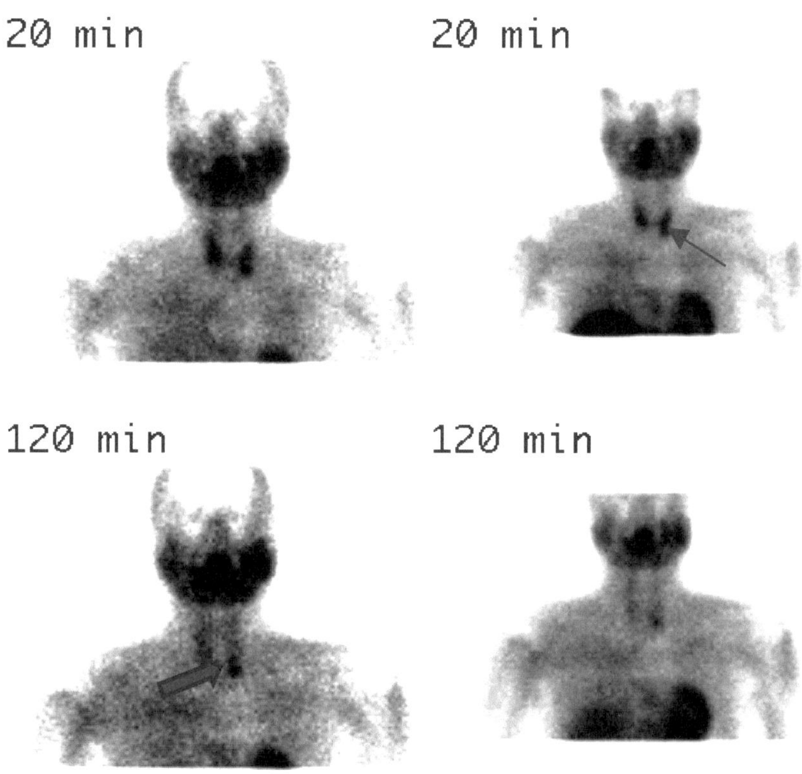

Figure 2.
Single-isotope dual-phase scintigraphy with ^{99m}Tc-sestamibi. On the early images (20 min) relatively diffuse uptake in the area of the thyroid gland and a focus of increased accumulation of the radionuclide (thin arrow), caudally of the left thyroid lobe are seen. On the late phase images (120 min) only a focus of a residual activity (thick arrow), caudally of the left thyroid lobe is visualized-suggesting adenoma of the lower left parathyroid gland.

In some cases, the obtained early and late images show no signs of abnormal accumulation of radionuclide, but when combined with SPECT, than adenomas located at the back of the thyroid gland become visible (**Figure 3a** and **b**).

So, the combination of a single-isotope dual-phase scintigraphy with ^{99m}Tc-sestamibi with SPECT can be of great help.

During many years in the past, two-dimensional images have been obtained, mainly AP-images, and rarely this was combined with lateral and oblique images [52, 53].

SPECT has gained more importance, because it gives three-dimensional images. There are accumulating data from the literature, that it improves sensitivity for discovering and localizing the hyperfunctioning parathyroid glands [54, 55]. The main reason for this is the improved contrast resolution of SPECT (**Figure 4**).

4.2.2 Single-isotope dual-phase scintigraphy with ^{99m}Tc-tetrofosmin

^{99m}Tc-tetrofosmin, another myocardial perfusion agent, is also used for parathyroid scintigraphy, but there are limited data in the literature for its use. Several

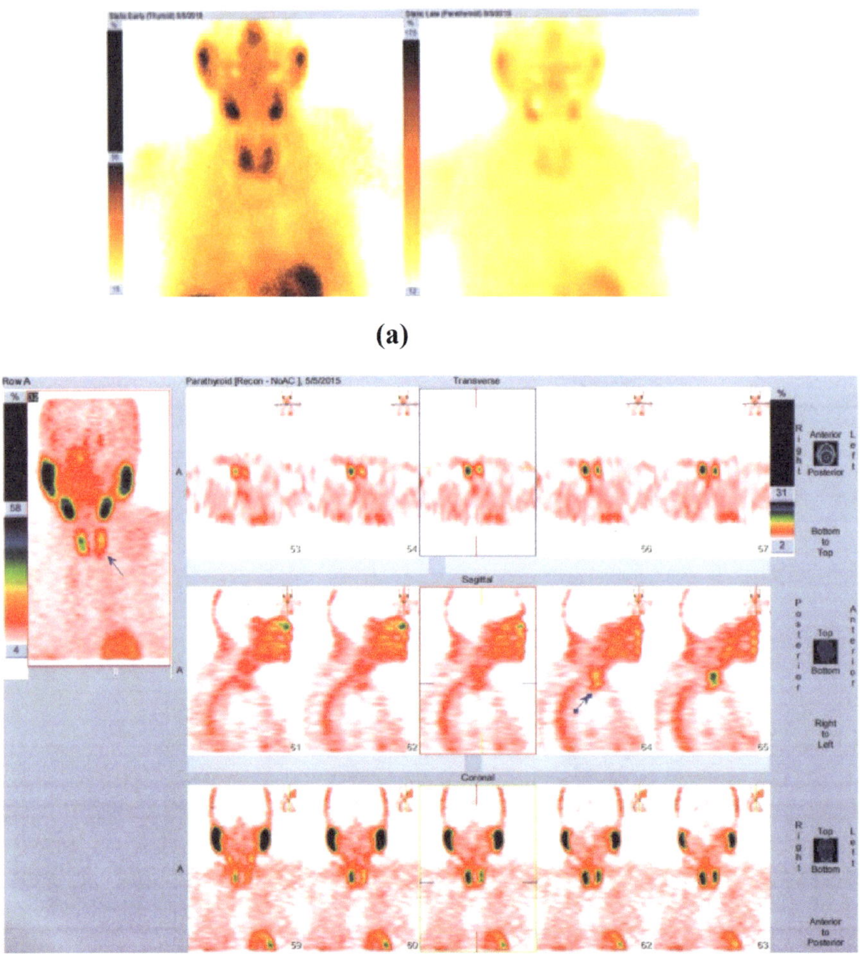

Figure 3.
(a) Single-isotope dual-phase scintigraphy with ^{99m}Tc-sestamibi. Early planar images show diffuse uptake in the thyroid gland. Late planar images show no sign of a focus of residual activity in the neck area or mediastinum. (b) (The same patient) ^{99m}Tc-sestamibi SPECT images show an area of a residual activity, located dorsally and caudally of the left thyroid lobe (arrows) suspicious for a parathyroid adenoma.

studies [26, 27] assess the diagnostic value of ^{99m}Tc-tetrofosmin scintigraphy for topic localization of the hyperfunctioning parathyroid glands in patients with PHPT. They show that this method was useful for the clinical practice and that the accumulation of ^{99m}Tc-tetrofosmin depended on the weight of the tumor and the level of PTH. The early images (15th min) prove to be better than the late ones (120th min). ^{99m}Tc-tetrofosmin is washed out more slowly from the thyroid gland than ^{99m}Tc-sestamibi but both radionuclides give better results in comparison with ^{99m}Tc-pertechnetate/^{201}Tl-substractional technique [56]. ^{99m}Tc-tetrofosmin looks promising alternative of ^{99m}Tc-sestamibi with similar properties and capabilities of localizing parathyroid adenomas.

Dual-isotope substractional scintigraphy with ^{99m}Tc-tetrofosmin/^{99m}Tc-pertechnetate and SPECT represent highly sensitive method for localization of parathyroid adenomas and their combination can further improve the diagnostic precision [57]. ^{99m}Tc-tetrofosmin, like ^{99m}Tc-sestamibi is not perfect for localization of hyperplastic parathyroid glands in patients with SHPT, because of its lower sensitivity [56]. ^{99m}Tc-tetrofosmin has some similarities with ^{99m}Tc-sestamibi, but its mechanism of accumulation in the cells is different. In contrast with ^{99m}Tc-sestamibi, which accumulation depends on mitochondria's membrane potential, retention of ^{99m}Tc-tetrofosmin depends mainly on cell's membrane potential [25]. ^{99m}Tc-tetrofosmin, shows slower wash out from the thyroid on the late planar images (120 min). This leads to the necessity to obtain additional later planar images—between 150 and 160 min. This slower wash out makes ^{99m}Tc-tetrofosmin to be unsuitable for performing single-isotope, dual-phase scintigraphy [25]. To avoid misleading, because of prolonged retention of the radiopharmaceutical in the thyroid adenomas, an US examination should be performed, especially in iodine deficient areas [56].

Figure 5 is presented a single-isotope dual-phase scintigraphy with ^{99m}Tc-tetrofosmin, combined with SPECT in a patient with PHPT.

In ^{99m}Tc-tetrofosmin scintigraphy early images at 20th min show better quality than the later ones at 120th min (**Figure 6a–c**).

Late planar images (120 min)—negative scan.

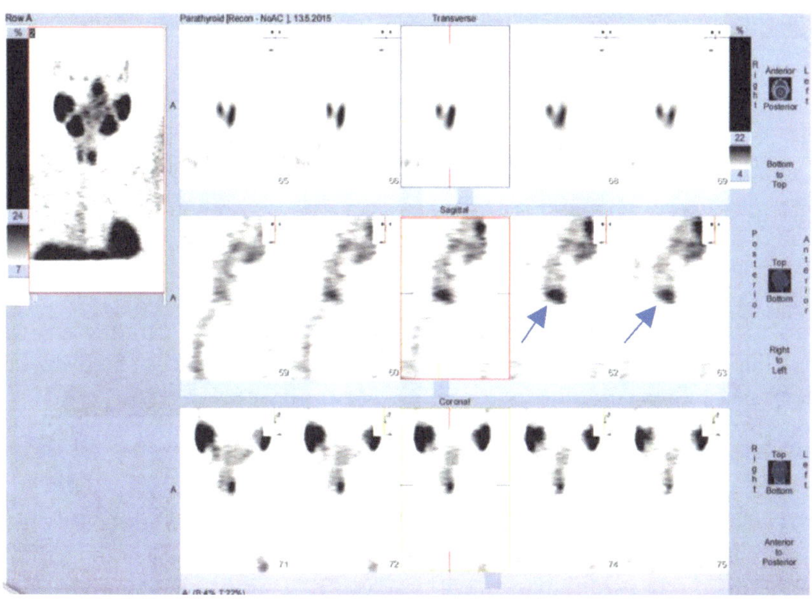

Figure 4.
Early ^{99m}Tc-sestamibi SPECT images showing an area of radionuclide accumulation (arrows), located dorsally and caudally of the left thyroid lobe.

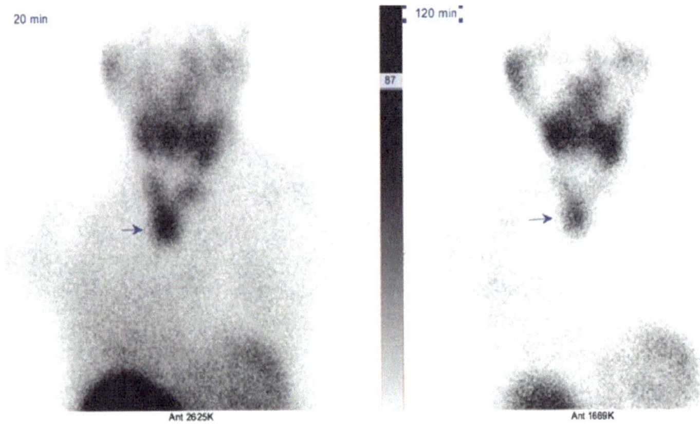

(a)

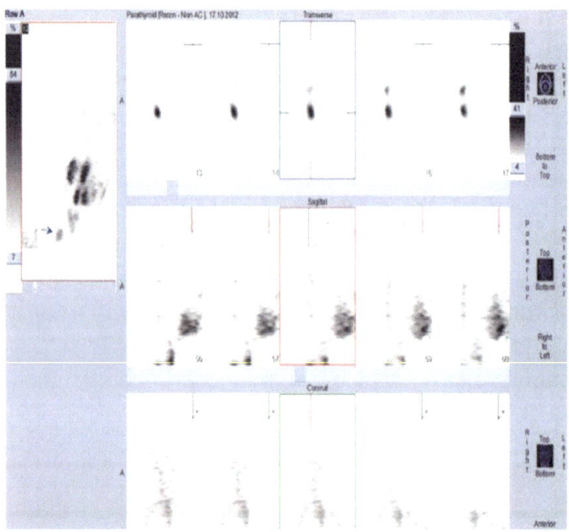

(b)

Figure 5.
(a) Early phase image (20 min) shows an intense uptake of the radionuclide at the lower part of the right thyroid lobe, which activity is still present on the late image (120 min) (arrows) and (b) (same patient) SPECT images showing an intense uptake dorsally and caudally of the right thyroid lob (arrow), suggestive for adenoma of the right lower parathyroid gland.

In this case, early SPECT gives opportunity to visualize adenomas, which were not seen on the late planar images, which is probably due to the rapid wash out of the radiopharmaceutical from some adenomas, as well as to the small sizes of the adenomas. When combined with SPECT, dual-phase scintigraphy with ^{99m}Tc-tetrofosmin can detect adenomas with rapid wash out of the radiopharmaceuticals.

Pearls/pitfalls:

a. The single isotope dual-phase scintigraphy with ^{99m}Tc-sestamibi or ^{99m}Tc-tetrofosmin could miss parathyroid adenomas with rapid washout of the radionuclide. The combination with early SPECT improves sensitivity.

b. The single isotope dual-phase scintigraphy with ^{99m}Tc-tetrofosmin in patients with PHPT and SHPT is with less sensitivity and specificity, because of the poor quality of the obtained images and slower washout of the radionuclide from the thyroid gland.

c. SPECT combined with single-isotope scintigraphy and subtractional methods for visualization of hyperfunctioning parathyroid adenomas in patients with PHPT and SHPT is a reliable additional modality. It does not cause additional and unnecessary exposure of the patients to the gamma-rays and can increase sensitivity.

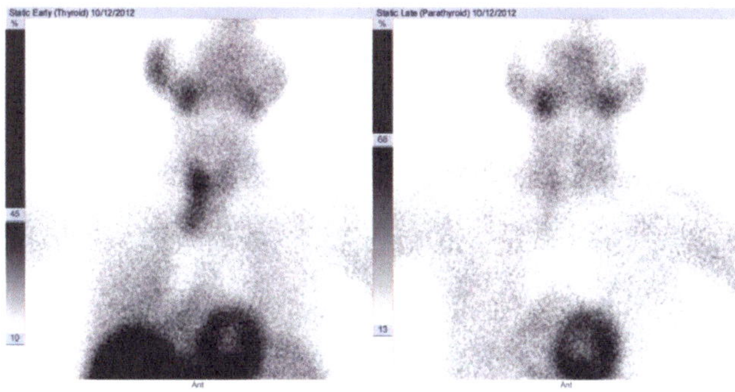

(a)

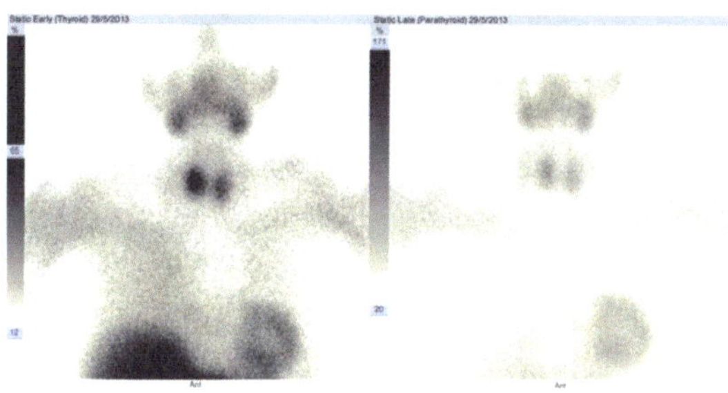

(b)

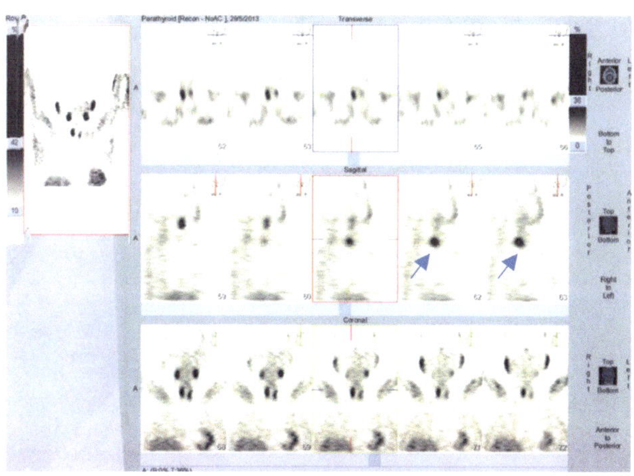

(c)

Figure 6.
(a) Single-isotope dual-phase scintigraphy with ^{99m}Tc-tetrofosmin. Early planar images (20 min) are with better quality, (b) (same patient) single-isotope dual-phase scintigraphy with ^{99m}Tc-tetrofosmin and (c) ^{99m}Tc-tetrofosmin SPECT images—an area (arroes) with high uptake located dorsally of the lower right lobe is seen, consistent with adenoma of the right lower parathyroid gland.

4.3 Dual-isotope subtractional scintigraphy with: ^{99m}Tc-pertehnetat/^{99m}Tc sestamibi or ^{99m}Tc-pertehnetat/^{99m}Tc-tetrofosmin

4.3.1 Dual-isotope subtractional scintigraphy with ^{99m}Tc-pertehnetat/^{99m}Tc sestamibi

The rationale that stands behind dual-isotope subtractional scintigraphy with ^{99m}Tc-pertehnetat/^{99m}Tc sestamibi, is that ^{99m}Tc-sestamibi accumulates in both, thyroid gland and hyperfunctioning parathyroid glands, while ^{99m}Tc-pertechnetate uptakes only in the thyroid. First thyroid specific radionuclide ^{99m}Tc-pertechnetate

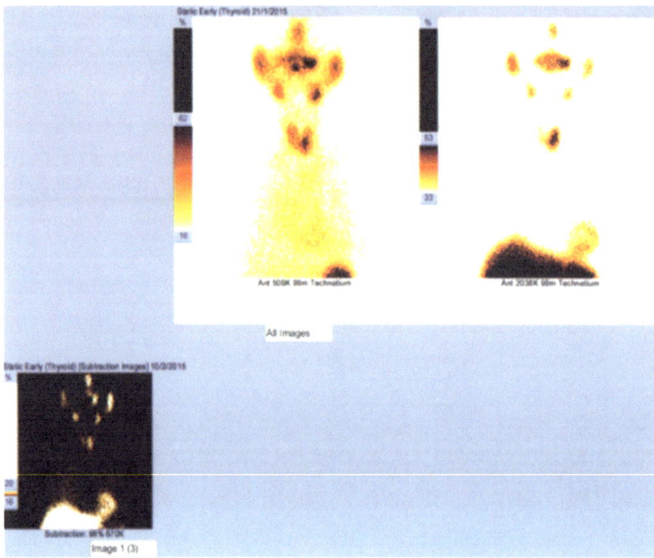

(a)

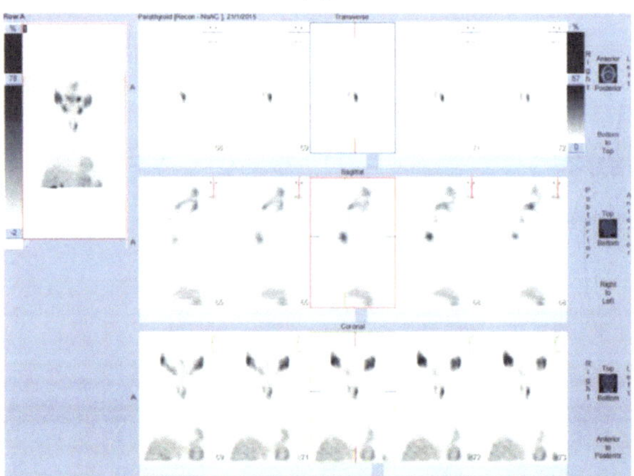

(b)

Figure 7.
(a) Dual-isotope subtractional scintigraphy with ^{99m}Tc-pertehnetat/^{99m}Tc sestamibi. Upper image on the left-image of thyroid gland obtained with ^{99m}Tc-pertehnetat. Upper image on the right an image obtained with ^{99m}Tc sestamibi (arrow). Lower image. Subtractional image showing a focus of a residual activity (arrow) in upper back part of the left thyroid lobe consistent with left parathyroid adenoma and (b) (same patient) dual-isotope subtractional scintigraphy with ^{99m}Tc-pertehnetat/^{99m}Tc sestamibi. Early SPECT images showing an area of intense uptake located dorsally and cranially of the left thyroid lobe.

is injected and at 30th min images are obtained. Afterwards, while the patient is still under the detector, second radionuclide ^{99m}Tc sestamibi with dual accumulation is applied and a second set of images on the 20th min are obtained. Later images are subtracted digitally from the first set of images and if a focus of residual activity on the subtractional images is detected, a hyperfunctioning parathyroid gland is supposed. The combination with early SPECT can improve sensitivity (**Figure 7a** and **b**).

The subtraction could be of help, when the patients had undergone surgery of the thyroid, but some thyroid parenchyma is still present. This method is important in the presence of more than one abnormal parathyroid gland.

Dual-isotope subtractional scintigraphy with ^{99m}Tc-pertehnetat/^{99m}Tc sestamibi combined with SPECT in a 51 years old man with MEN-type 1

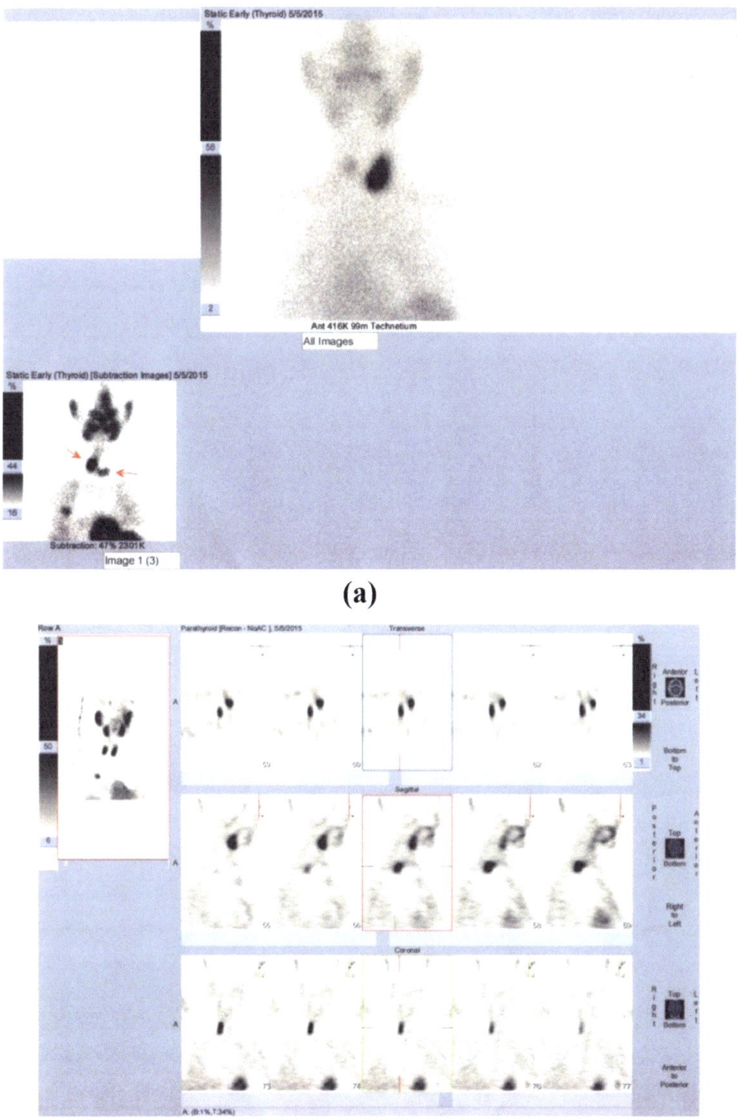

(a)

(b)

Figure 8.
(a) Dual-isotope subtractional scintigraphy with ^{99m}Tc-pertehnetat/^{99m}Tc sestamibi. Subtractional image showing two areas of intense uptake consistent with two parathyroid adenomas and (b) SPECT images showing an area of intense uptake located dorsally and caudally of the right thyroid lobe.

syndrome—pheochromocytoma, parathyroid adenoma and prolactinoma, who had previously undergone thyroid (subtotal thyroidectomy) and parathyroid (left upper parathyroid gland) surgery. Subtractional images (**Figure 8a**) and early SPECT images (**Figure 8b**) show two areas of intense uptake located below the remnants of the both thyroid lobes. SPECT images show that the lesion below the right thyroid lobe was located also adjacent to the back part of the right thyroid lobe.

In some cases, obtaining late images could also be of help. Combining dual-isotope, ^{99m}Tc-pertehnetat/^{99m}Tc sestamibi, subtractional scintigraphy with SPECT, and also recording late planar images on the 120th min (late phase) would improve sensitivity (**Figures 9** and **10**).

Pearls/pitfalls

a. Dual isotope subtractional scintigraphy with ^{99m}Tc-pertehnetat/^{99m}Tc sestamibi or ^{99m}Tc-pertehnetat/^{99m}Tc-tetrofosmin allows visualization of abnormal parathyroid glands after subtraction is performed, even on the early obtained images.

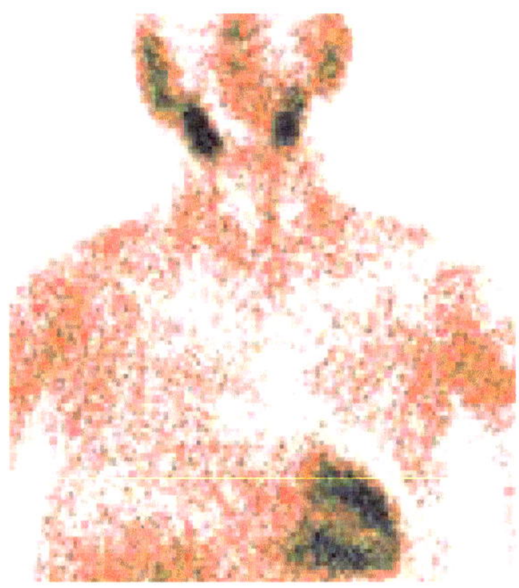

(a)

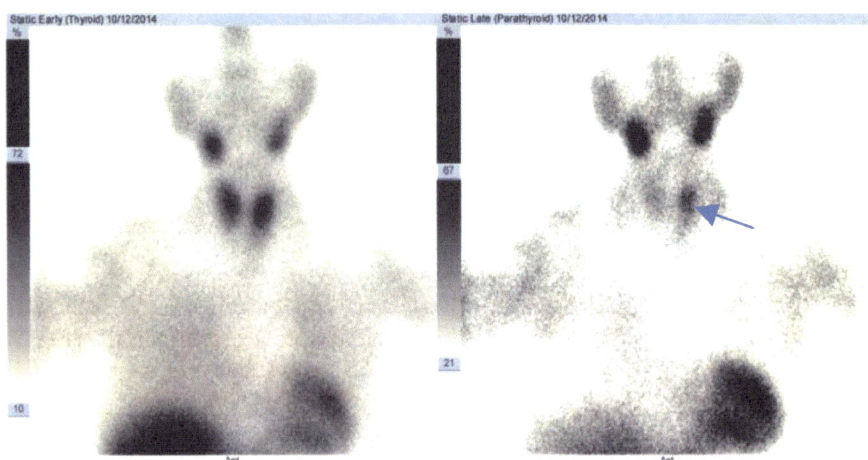

(b)

Figure 9.
(a) Dual-isotope subtractional scintigraphy with ^{99m}Tc-pertehnetat/^{99m}Tc sestamibi. Subtractional image showing no residual activity in the areas of the neck and chest and (b) late planar images showing a residual activity (arrow) in the middle of the left thyroid lobe, consistent with left parathyroid adenoma.

This helps to shorten the time of examination to 80–90 min and is of great use in the postsurgical follow up and when more than one abnormal gland is present.

b. Disadvantages of the subtractional scintigraphy with ^{99m}Tc-pertehnetat/^{99m}Tc sestamibi or ^{99m}Tc-pertehnetat/^{99m}Tc-tetrofosmin are: necessity of applying of two radionuclides, the need of very precise positioning of the patients in this dual phase method requiring full collaboration from patient's side and the probability of the presence of artifacts in the obtained images.

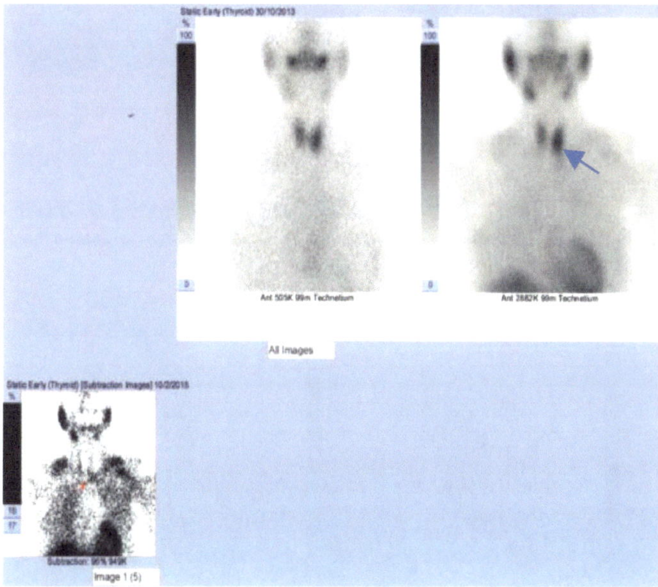

(a)

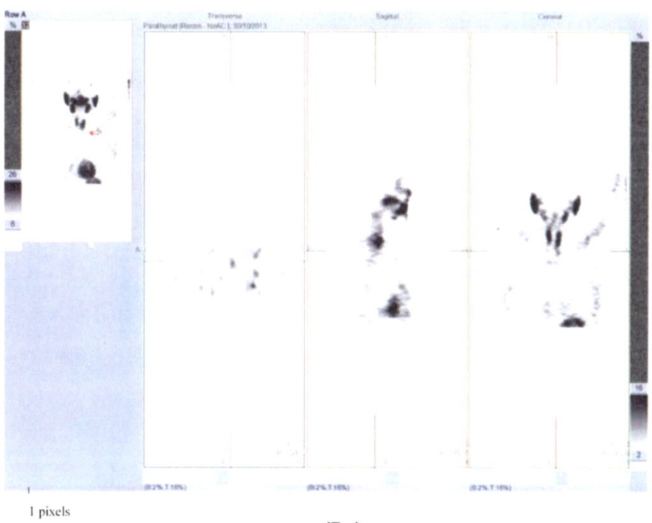

(b)

Figure 10.
(a) Dual-isotope subtractional method with ^{99m}Tc-pertehnetat/^{99m}Tc-tetrofosmin. The upper row: on the left image of the thyroid gland with ^{99m}Tc-pertehnetat and on the right image of the parathyroid gland with ^{99m}Tc-tetrofosmin (arrow). The lower row shows subtractional image representing adenoma of left parathyroid gland and (b) dual-isotope subtractional method with ^{99m}Tc-pertehnetat/^{99m}Tc-tetrofosmin early SPECT images showing an area of hyper fixation, located caudally of the left thyroid lobe.

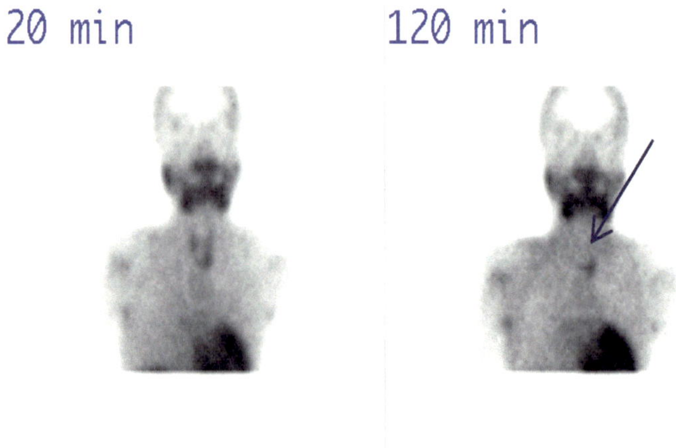

Figure 11.
Single-isotope, dual-phase scintigraphy with ^{99m}Tc-sestamibi in a patient with secondary hyperparathyroidism. The late phase (120 min) show a focus of residual activity (arrow)—consistent with parathyroid adenoma (probably tertiary hyperparathyroidism).

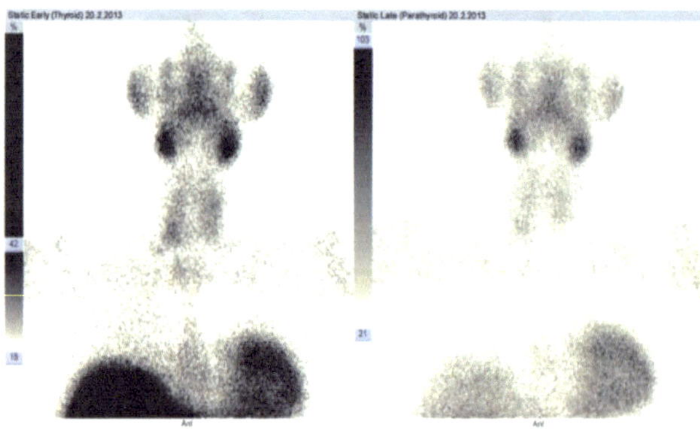

(a)

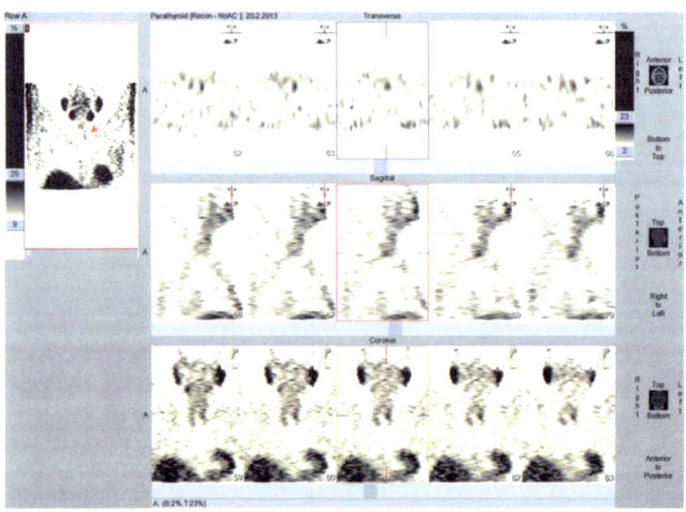

(b)

Figure 12.
(a) Single-isotope, dual-phase scintigraphy with ^{99m}Tc-tetrofosmin in a patient with secondary hyperparathyroidism. Early (20 min) and late (120 min) images show no focus of a residual activity in the area of neck and mediastinum and (b) (same patient) early SPECT images showing an area of nuclide accumulation caudally of the left thyroid lobe, suspicious for parathyroid adenoma.

4.4 Secondary hyperparathyroidism

Secondary hyperparathyroidism is characterized with hyperplasia of parathyroid glands, because it is caused by longstanding uncontrolled hypocalcemia, which leads to a profound overstimulation of a previously normal parathyroid glands. Over time this overstimulation causes hyperplasia and eventually adenomatous changes (tertiary hyperparathyroidism) of the parathyroid glands with PTH levels far more exceeding those observed in PHPT (**Figure 11**). Nevertheless, hyperplastic parathyroid glands usually show faster wash out of the radionuclides in comparison to solitary adenomas, which makes them more difficult to be visualized with scintigraphy (**Figure 12**). Negative scans, may be associated with the possible suppression of the accumulation of radiopharmaceuticals in the parathyroid cells as a result of the concomitant calcitriol intake. The use of calcium channel blockers may affect the uptake of ^{99m}Tc-sestamibi by parathyroid cells and reduce the sensitivity of the method. A study found that negative scans are twice as likely in patients taking calcium antagonists than those who do not take these medications (OR2, 88.95% CI, 1.03–8.10, p 0.045) [58]. So, adding the poor general condition of the patients, pathologically changed parathyroid glands are more difficult to be localized in SHPT than in PHPT.

5. Conclusions

The visualization of abnormal parathyroid glands is difficult due to their variations in number and localization. Noninvasive parathyroid imaging studies include ^{99m}Tc-sestamibi scintigraphy, ultrasonography, computed tomography scanning, magnetic resonance imaging, and positron emission tomography. There is a general consensus that the most sensitive and specific imaging modality is the scintigraphy with ^{99m}Tc-sestamibi or ^{99m}Tc-tetrofosmin. ^{99m}Tc-sestamibi scintigraphy significantly increases the role of preoperative scintigraphy in patients with hyperparathyroidism and allows unilateral surgical approach with minimally invasive parathyroidectomy to be used. Generally three protocols with the use of two radiopharmaceuticals, ^{99m}Tc-sestamibi or ^{99m}Tc-tetrofosmin, are most widely applied: single-phase dual-isotope subtraction, dual-phase single-isotope and combination of both. Each one of them has specific advantages and disadvantages. While, single parathyroid adenomas are localized with greater precision, hyperfunctioning parathyroid hyperplastic cells represent a real challenge to the imaging modalities.

Several factors can influence the radionuclide uptake in pathologically changed parathyroid cells:

a. biochemical factors

- Total calcium levels—higher preoperative calcium levels are more frequently seen in patients with positive scans.

- Parathyroid hormone levels.

- A significant correlation between radiopharmaceutical uptake and preoperative levels of PTH is observed. As higher PTH is, as higher is the possibility for positive scans.

- Vitamin D levels.

- Patents with vitamin D deficiency are more likely to have positive scans.

- Suboptimal levels of vitamin D, can stimulate the growth of the parathyroid adenomas independently from hypocalcemia and 1,25-dihydroxyvitamin D_3 deficit can change the set-point of calcium suppressive effect upon PTH secretion [59].

- Calcium-channel blockers.

- The use of calcium-channel blockers can influence the uptake of the radiopharmaceutical in the parathyroid cells diminishing the sensitivity of the method.

b. biological factors

- Size—although considered to be very important, it is not the only determining factor.

- Type of cells of the parathyroid adenoma—because oxyphilic cells contain more mitochondria, they uptake radionuclides to a larger extent.

- P glycoprotein and MDR gene products.

Uptake of ^{99m}Tc-sestamibi and ^{99m}Tc-tetrofosmin in the cells of the parathyroid adenomas depends on the activity of the P glycoprotein coded by MDR gene, which is functioning as an ATP dependent efflux pump, protecting against accumulation of lipophilic cationic radiopharmaceuticals, including ^{99m}Tc-tetrofosmin [60]. The expression of P glycoprotein in the parathyroid adenomas appears to be important factor determining radiopharmaceutical uptake. In one study 71% (10 out of 14) of adenomas with high P glycoprotein membrane activity have shown negative scans, 70% (45 out of 64) with negative P glycoprotein expression ($p = 0.006$) have shown positive scans [61].

Author details

Albena Dimitrova Botushanova[1] and Nikolay Petrov Botushanov[2]*

1 Department of Clinical Oncology, Section of Radiotherapy and Nuclear Medicine, Medical University-Plovdiv, UMHAT "St. George" EAD, Bulgaria

2 Second Department of Internal Diseases, Section of Endocrinology and Metabolic Diseases, Medical University-Plovdiv, MHAT "Medline Clinic" AD, Bulgaria

*Address all correspondence to: nbotush@gmail.com

IntechOpen

© 2019 The Author(s). Licensee IntechOpen. This chapter is distributed under the terms of the Creative Commons Attribution License (http://creativecommons.org/licenses/by/3.0), which permits unrestricted use, distribution, and reproduction in any medium, provided the original work is properly cited.

References

[1] Kearns AE, Thompson GB. Medical and surgical management of hyperparathyroidism. Mayo Clinic Proceedings. 2002;**77**(1):87-91

[2] Taniegra ED. Hyperparathyroidism. American Family Physician. 2004;**69**(2):333-339

[3] Ruda JM, Hollenbeak C, Stack BC Jr. A systematic review of the diagnosis and treatment of primary hyperparathyroidism from 1995 to 2003. Otolaryngology and Head and Neck Surgery. 2005;**132**(3):359-372

[4] Russell CF, Laird JD, Ferguson WR. Scan-directed unilateral cervical exploration for parathyroid adenoma: A legitimate approach? World Journal of Surgery. 1990;**14**(3):406-409

[5] Hansberger HR, Osborn AG, Ross J, Macdonald A. Thyroid gland and parathyroid glands. In: Diagnostic and Surgical Imaging Anatomy: Brain, Head and Neck, Spine. Amirsys: Salt Lake City, Utah. p. 2006

[6] Dufour DR, Wilkerson SY. Factors related to parathyroid weight in normal persons. Archives of Pathology & Laboratory Medicine. 1983;**107**(4):167-172

[7] Phitayakorn R, McHenry CR. Incidence and location of ectopic abnormal parathyroid glands. American Journal of Surgery. 2006;**191**(3):418-423

[8] Pellitteri PK, Sofferman RA, Randolph GW. Surgical management of parathyroid disorders. In: Cummings CW, Haughey BH, Thomas JR, Harker LA, Flint PW, editors. Cummings Otolaryngology: Head and Neck Surgery. 4th ed. Philadelphia Pa: Mosby; 2005

[9] DeLellis RA. Surgical pathology of the parathyroid glands. In: Randolph G, editor. Surgery of the Thyroid and Parathyroid Glands. St. Louis, MO: Elsevier; 2003. pp. 571-577

[10] De Feo MI, Colagrande S, Biagini C, Tonarei A, Vaggelli L, et al. Parathyroid glands: Combination of (99m)Tc MIBI scintigraphy and US for demonstration of parathyroid glands and nodules. Radiology. 2000;**241**(2):393-402

[11] Waldorf JC, van Heerden JA, Gorman CA, Grant CS, Wahner HW. (^{75}Se) Selenomethionine scanning for parathyroid localization should be abandoned. Mayo Clinic Proceedings. 1984;**59**:534-537

[12] Van Husen R, Kim LT. Accuracy of surgeon performed ultrasound in parathyroid localization. World Journal of Surgery. 2004:1122-1126

[13] Mortenson ME, Evans DB Hunter GJ, et al. Parathyroid exploration in the reoperative neck: Improved preoperative localization with 4D-computer tomography. Journal of the American College of Surgeons. 2008;**206**:888-895

[14] Dugonjic S, Ajdinovic B, Cerovic S, Jankovic Z. Validity of dual tracer 99mTc-tetrofosmin and Tc-pertechnetate sultraction parathyroid scintigraphy in patients with primary and secondary hyperparathyroidism. Vojnosanitetski Pregled. 2009;**66**(12):949-953

[15] Krausz Y, Horne T, Wynchank S, Halevy A. Lateral neck imaging for spatial localization of parathyroid tissue. Nuclear Medicine and Biology. 1995;**22**(3):394

[16] Bergenfelz A, Tennvall J, Valdermarsson S, Lindblom P, Tibblin S. Sestamibi versus thallium subtraction scintigraphy in parathyroid localization: A prospective comparative study in patients with predominantly mild

primary hyperparathyroidism. Surgery. 1997;**121**(6):601-605

[17] Coakley AJ, Kettle AG, Wells CP, O'Doherty MJ, Collins RE. 99mTc-sestamibi—A new agent for parathyroid imaging. Nuclear Medicine Communications. 1989;**10**(11):791-794

[18] Weber CJ, Vansant J, Alazraki N. Value of technetium 99m sestamibi/ iodine 123 imaging in reoperative parathyroid surgery. Surgery. 1993;**114**(6):1011-1018

[19] Bhatnagar A, Vezza PR, Bryan JA, Atkins FB, Ziessman HA. Technetium 99m sestamibi parathyroid scintigraphy: Effect of P-glycoprotein, histology and tumor size on detectability. Journal of Nuclear Medicine. 1998;**39**:1617-1620

[20] Chudzinski W, Niderla J, Lasiecka Z, Wilczynski G, Gornicka B, Wasiutynshi A, et al. P-glycoprotein expression influences the result of 99mTc-MIBI scintigraphy in tertiary hyperparathyroidism. International Journal of Molecular Medicine. 2005;**16**:215-219

[21] Grzela T, Chudzinski W, Lazarczyk M, Niderla J, Dziunycz P, Milewski L, et al. Persisted/recurrent hyperparathyroidism associated with development of multi-drug resistance phenotype and proliferation of parathyroid transplants. International Journal of Molecular Medicine. 2004;**14**:559-599

[22] Taillefer R, Boucher Y, Potvin C, Lambert R. Detection and localization of parathyroid adenomas in patients with hyperparathyroidism using a single radionuclide imaging procedure with technetium-99m-sestamibi (double-phase study). Journal of Nuclear Medicine. 1992;**33**(10):1801-1807

[23] Grzela T, Chudzinski W, Lasiecka Z, Niderla J, Wilczynski G, Gornicka B, et al. The calcium-sensing receptor and vitamin D receptor expression in tertiary hyperparathyroidism. International Journal of Molecular Medicine. 2006;**17**:1801-1807

[24] Casara D, Rubello D, Piotto A, Pelizzo MR. ^{99m}Tc-MIBI radio-guided minimally invasive parathyroid surgery planned on the basis of a preoperative combined ^{99m}Tc-pertechnetate/^{99m}Tc-MiBi and altrasound imaging protocol. European Journal of Nuclear Medicine. 2000;**27**:1300-1304

[25] Froberg AC, Valkema R, Bonjer HJ, Krenning EP. ^{99m}Tc-tetrofosmin or ^{99m}Tc sestamibi for double-phase parathyroid scintigraphy? European Journal of Nuclear Medicine and Molecular Imaging. 2003;**30**:193-196

[26] Hiromatsu Y, Ishibashi M, Nishida H, Okuda S, Miyake I. Technetium-99m tetrofosmin parathyroid imaging in patients with primary hyperparathyroidism. Internal Medicine. 2000;**39**(2):101-106

[27] Vallejos V, Martin-Comin J, Gonzalez MT, Rafecas R, Munoz A, Fernandez A, et al. The usefulness of Tc-99m tetrofosmin scintigraphy in the diagnosis and localization of hyperfunctioning parathyroid glands. Clinical Nuclear Medicine. 1999;**24**(12):959-964

[28] Palestro CJ, Tomas MB, Tronco GG. Radionuclide imaging of the parathyroid glands. Seminars in Nuclear Medicine. 2005;**35**(4):266-276

[29] Standrock D, Merino MJ, Norton JA, Neumann RD. Parathyroid imaging by Tc/Tl scintigraphy. European Journal of Nuclear Medicine. 1990;**16**(8-10):607-613

[30] Liehn JC, Delisle MJ, Flamen JB. Improvement of parathyroid Tl-Tc scintigraphy by using a new image subtraction method. European Journal of Nuclear Medicine. 1988;**14**(4):184-189

[31] Rauth JD, Sessions RB, Shupe SC, Ziessman HA. Comprasion of Tc-99m MIBI and Tl-201/Tc-99m pertechnetate for diagnosis of primary hyperparathyroidism. Clinical Nuclear Medicine. 1996;**21**(8):602-608

[32] 62.Leslie WD, Dupont JO, Bybel B, Riese KT. Parathyroid 99mTc-sestamibi scintigraphy: Dual-traser subtraction in superior to double-phase washout. European Journal of Nuclear Medicine and Molecular Imaging. 2002;**29**(12):1566-1570

[33] As A, Koizumi K, Toyama K, Araki T. Uptake of technetium-99m-tetrofosmin, technetium-99m-MIBI and thallium-201 in tumor cell lines. Journal of Nuclear Medicine. 1996;**37**(10):1551-1556

[34] O'Donety MJ, Kettle AG, Wells CP, et al. Parathyroid imaging with technetium-99m-sestamibi:preoperative localization and tissue uptake studies. Journal of Nuclear Medicine. 1998;**33**:313-318

[35] Lee VS, Spritzer CE, Coleman RE, Wilkinson RHJ, Coogan AC, Leight GSJ. The complementary roles of fast spin-echo MR imaging and duble-phase 99m Tc-sestamibi scintigraphy for localization of hyperfunctioning parathyroid glans. American Journal of Roentgenology. 1996;**167**(6):1555-1562

[36] Moka D, Voth E, Dietlein M, et al. Technetium 99m-MIBI-SPECT: A higly sensitive diagnostic tool for localization of parathyroid adenomas. Surgery. 2000;**128**(1):29-35

[37] Casara D, Rubello D, Piotto D, Pelizzo MR. 99mTc-MIBI radio-guided minimally invasive parathyroid surgery planned on the basis of a preoperative combined 99mTc-pertechnetate/99mTc-MIBI and ultrasound imaging protocol. European Journal of Nuclear Medicine. 2000;**27**(9):1300-1304

[38] Melliere D, Hindie E, Voisin MC, et al. Primary hyperthyroidism. Optimization of surgical results with systematic preoperative 99mTc-sestamibi scintigraphy. Chirurgie. 1997;**122**(2):98-104

[39] Pons F, Torregrosa JV, Vidal-Sicart S, Sabater L, Fuster D, Fernandez-Cruz L, et al. Preoperative parathyroid gland localization with 99Tc-sestamibi in secondary hyperparathyroidism. European Journal of Nuclear Medicine. 1997;**24**(12):1494-1498

[40] Ishibashi M, Nishida H, Okuda S, Suekane S. Localization of parathyroid glands in hemodialysis patients using Tc-99m Sestamibi imaging. Nephron. 1998;**78**:48

[41] Walgenbach S, Dutkowski P, Andreas J, Bockisch A, Junginger T. 99mT-MIBI-scintigraphy before parathyroid surgery? Zentralblatt für Chirurgie. 2000;**124**(3):214-219

[42] Mimura Y, Kanauchi H, Ogawa T, Kammori M, Kaminishi M. Review of 41 patients operated on for primary hyperparathyroidism. Biomedicine & Pharmacotherapy. 2000;**54** (Suppl. 1):72-76

[43] Piga M, Bolasco P, Satta L, Altieri P, Loi G, Nicolosi A, et al. MariottiDouble phase parathyroid technetium-99m-MIBI scintigraphy to identify functional autonomy in secondary hyperparathyroidism. Journal of Nuclear Medicine. 1996;**37**(4):565-569

[44] Torregrosa JV. Usefulness of double-phase technetium-99m sestamibi scintigraphy in secondary hyperparathyroidism before parathyroidetomy. Journal of Nuclear Medicine. 1999;**40**:1434-1440

[45] Kusakabe K, Oshima M, Takami H, Murata H, Aburano T, Kabo A. Evaluation of clinical utility of 99mTc-MIBI scintigraphy

in localization of hyperfunctioning parathyroid lesions in patients with hyperparathyroidism—A report of multicenter phase 3 clinical trials. Kaku Igaku. 1998;**35**(9):887-899

[46] Rothmund H, Diethelm J, Brunner C, et al. Diagnosis and surgical treatment of mediastinal parathyroid tumors. Annals of Surgery. 1976;**183**:139-145

[47] Rubello D, Mazzarollo R, Casara D. The role of technetium-99m sestamibi scintigraphy in the planning of therapy and follow-up of patient with differentiated thyroid carcinoma after surgery. European Journal of Nuclear Medicine. 2000;**27**(4):431-440

[48] Benard F, Lefebre B, Beuvon F, Langlois MF, Bisson G. Rapid washout of technetium-99-MIBI from a large parathyroid adenoma. Journal of Nuclear Medicine. 1995;**36**(2):241-243

[49] Hung GU, Wu HS, Tsai SC, Kao CH, et al. Recurrent hyperfunctioning in parathyroid gland demonstratedon radionuclide imaging and an intraoperative gamma probe. Clinical Nuclear Medicine. 2000;**25**(5):348-350

[50] Lomonte C, Buonvino N, Selvaggiolo M, Dassira M, Grasso G, Vernaglione L, et al. Sestamibi scintigraphy, topography, and histopathology of paratjyroid glands in secondary hyperparathyroidism. American Journal of Kidney Diseases. 2006;**48**(4):638-644

[51] Olaizola I, Zingrafe J, Heuguerot C, Fajardo L, Leger A, et al. 99mTc-Sestamibi parathyroid scintigraphy in chronic haemodialysis patients: Static and dynamic explorations. Nephrology, Dialysis, Transplantation. 2000;**15**(8):1201-1206

[52] Krausz Y, Horne T, Wynchank S, Halevy A. Lateral neec imaging for spatial localization of parathyroid tissue. Nuclear Medicine and Biology. 1995;**22**(3):394

[53] ArveschougAK,BertelsenH,VammenB, Brochner-Mortensen J. Preoperative dual-phase parathyroid imaging with Tc-99m-sestamibi: Accuracy and reproducibility of pinhole collimator with and without oblique images. Clinical Nuclear Medicine. 2007;**32**(1):9-12

[54] Moka D, Voth E, Dietlein M, Larena-Avellaneda A, Schicha H. Technetium 99m-MIBI-SPECT: A highly sensitive diagnostic tool for localization of parathyroid adenomas. Surgery. 2000;**128**(1):29-35

[55] Lorberboym M, Minski I, Macadziob S, Nikolov G, Schachter P. Incremental diagnostic value of preoperative 99mTc-MIBI SPECT in patients with a parathyroid adenoma. Journal of Nuclear Medicine. 2003;**44**(6):904-908

[56] Gallowitsch HJ, Mikosch P, Kresnik E, Gomez I, Lind P. Technetium 99m tetrofosmin parathyroid imaging. Results with double-phase study and SPECT in primary and secondary hyperparathyroidism. Investigative Radiology. 1997;**32**(8):459-465

[57] Gallowitsch HJ, Mikosch P, Kresnik E, Unterweger O, Lind P. Comparison between 99mTc-tetrofosmin/pertechnetate subtraction scintigraphy and 99mTc-tetrofosmin SPECT for preoperative localization of parathyroid adenoma in an endemic goiter area. Investigative Radiology. 2000;**35**(8):453-459

[58] Friedman K, Somervell H, Patel P, Melton GB, Garrett-Mayer E, Dackiw AP, et al. Effect of calcium channel blockers on the sensitivity of pre-operative 99mTc-MIBI SPECT for hyperparathyroidism. Surgery. 2004;**136**(6):1199-1204

[59] Rao DS, Honasoge M, Divine GW, Phillips ER, Lee MW, Ansari MR, et al. Effect of vitamin D nutrition on parathyroid adenoma weight: Pathogenetic and clinical implications. The Journal of Clinical Endocrinology and Metabolism. 2000;**85**(3):1054-1058

[60] Piwnica-Worms D, Chiu ML, Budding M, Kronauge JF, Kramer RA, Croop JM. Functional imaging of multidrug-resistant P-glycoprotein with an organotechnetium complex. Cancer Research. 1993;**53**(5):977-984

[61] Gupta Y, Ahmed R, Happerfield L, Pinder SE, Balan KK, Wishart GC. P-glycoprotein expression is associated with sestamibi washout in primary hyperparathyroidism. The British Journal of Surgery. 2007;**94**(12):1491-1495

Section 2

Nuclear Medicine Mechanism Imaging and Therapy

Chapter 4

Theranostics: New Era in Nuclear Medicine and Radiopharmaceuticals

Chanchal Deep Kaur, Koushlesh Kumar Mishra, Anil Sahu, Rajnikant Panik, Pankaj Kashyap, Saraswati Prasad Mishra and Anand Kumar

Abstract

Malignancy and many inflammatory diseases have become a major concern for mankind over the years. The conventional therapy of these diseases lacks the effectiveness of the better diagnosis and targeted treatment of these diseases, but nuclear medicine can be regarded as a savior in the current scenario. Over the years, radioactivity of radioisotopes has been employed for treatment of many diseases. Nuclear medicines came up with radiopharmaceuticals that impart the ability to destroy specific diseased cells with high-energy-emitting radionuclides. Moreover, the emergence of theranostics, which is a combination of single drug used both for diagnostic as well as therapeutic purpose, has added a new feather in the field of nuclear medicines for providing a specific and personalized treatment to the patient. The current chapter discusses about techniques used for imaging of these radionuclides for better therapy and diagnosis of the root cause of the concerned disease by positron emission tomography (PET)/CT and single photon emission computed tomography (SPECT)/CT as well as the advantages and disadvantages associated with them. It also describes about applications of theranostics and nuclear imaging in cancer treatment and their future perspective.

Keywords: radionuclides, nuclear medicines, nuclear imaging, theranostics, radiopharmaceuticals

1. Introduction to radioisotopes and radiopharmaceuticals

Scientist has discovered that earth contains many elements with varying configuration. These elements with varying configuration are called isotopes. Isotopes are atoms with same atomic number with varying atomic weight. Isotopes can be divided into two parts depending on the ability to emit radiation. One that does not emit radiations is called stable isotopes and other are called unstable isotopes. Unstable isotopes emit radiations to achieve a more stable configuration. These are called as radioisotopes. Instability of radioisotopes is due to presence of unstable combination of neutron and proton in their atoms and nucleus contains excess of energy. This characteristic of radioisotopes can be natural or instability can be created artificially by changing the atoms. Naturally radioisotope is uranium-238 and it accounts to 0.7% of total naturally occurring isotopes. Artificial radioisotopes are fluorine and molybdenum which are produced artificially by using cyclotrons and nuclear reactors respectively. Presently there are around 3800 radioisotopes out of which 200 radioisotopes are being used. Among the isotopes that are used most of them are of artificial origin. Artificial radioisotopes are primarily made by two methods as mentioned above i.e. through nuclear reactor and by cyclotron. By nuclear reactor neutrons are introduced into the nucleus of atom whereas in case of cyclotron proton are introduced. To become stable radioisotopes emits alpha or beta particle along with electromagnetic radiation of gamma rays. This phenomenon is called as radioactive decay. These radioisotopes have variety of uses, when they are used in the field of pharmaceuticals they are termed as radiopharmaceuticals.

1.1 Radiopharmaceuticals

These are radioactive medicines that can be given by oral, intravenous or interstitial route to treat or diagnose malignancy. Administration of these drugs is done in the presence of specialist called radio pharmacist. These radioactive medicines have the ability to destroy cancerous cell by emitting radiation when it reaches its target cell. Radiopharmaceuticals for treatment and diagnosis of cancers associated with thyroid, brain, bones or lymphoma already been discovered.

In addition to treatment radiopharmaceuticals are also used for the purpose of diagnosis. The drugs used for diagnosis are called as tracers. The radiation of diagnostic radiopharmaceuticals is smaller as compared to radiation emitted by radiopharmaceuticals used for treatment. Radiopharmaceuticals are either single isotopes or sometimes the isotopes are combined with a kit [1]. The kit is prepackaging of ingredients which are sterile and are meant for preparation of radiopharmaceuticals. They are combination of substances such as antioxidant, buffer, reductant and ligands that are when combined with the radioisotopes produces the resultant product. Kits are very beneficial as they are not in contact with the outer environment so there is no chance of any contamination [2].

1.2 Technetium 99m

The isotope that is used for the purpose of labeling of kits used for diagnosis is technetium 99m abbreviated as 99mTc (**Figure 1**). It radiates only gamma radiation that is compatible with gamma camera. 99mTc also has the property of binding with the tracers. Advantage of technetium is that it has smaller biological half-life and better renal clearance for the unabsorbed radiopharmaceuticals that helps in getting a better quality of image from the absorbed ones. The dose of technetium depends on the kit, the organ on which it has to be used for imaging and on the test to be performed [3]. Determination of dose for children is very crucial as the cells

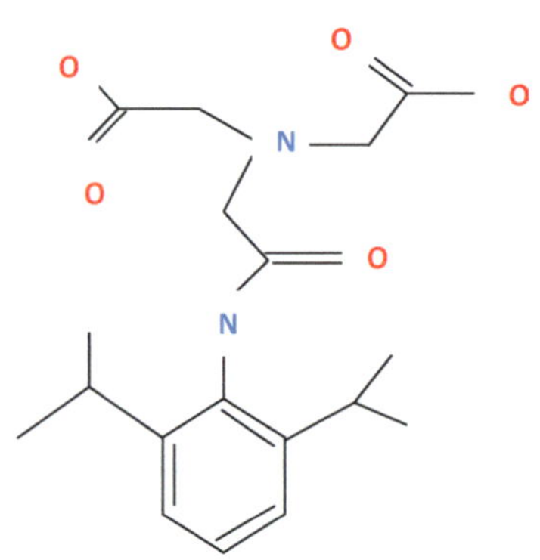

Figure 1.
Chemical structure of technetium 99m.

are in dividing states so sensitivity towards radiation can be higher, organ size body ratio also varies to greater extent in comparison with adult. So in case of children a balanced level of administration is required [4].

Different kit labeled with 99mTc used for imaging of different organs is mentioned below.

1.2.1 Bone

For detection of the areas that are metabolizing the bones kits with bisphosphonates are used. Scan of bone is done by injecting radiopharmaceuticals into the peripheral vein of patient and then after 3 h imaging is done so that within the three hours the bisphosphonates will get incorporated into the osteoblast cells.

1.2.2 Kidney

For the imaging of kidney, there are three radiopharmaceuticals, namely

i. Radiolabelled mercaptoacetyltriglycine (Mag-3; mertiatide)

ii. Radiolabelled diethylenetriaminepentaacetic acid (DTPA; pentetate)

iii. Radiolabelled dimercaptosuccinic acid (DMSA; succimer

Mag-3; mertiatide is used for the purpose of determining the blood flow to the kidney and for graphically presenting the renal function. Mag-3 has a clearance of 94% after 3 h that helps in getting better quality of image and the exposure of patient to the radiation is also lower. DTPA; pentetate is used to determining rate of glomerular filtration during chemotherapy of kidney. Lastly DMSA; succimer is used a tool for studying morphology of renal cortex and ectopic kidney.

1.2.3 Brain

Kit used for the check the blood flow within the brain after conditions like epilepsy, migraine or Alzheimer's disease or stroke of brain contains 99mTc-labeled exametazime. This is product of lipophilic origin without any charge on it and it penetrates better through blood brain barrier. It takes around one minute after injection for it to reach brain and up to 7% reaches the brain.

1.2.4 Heart

For cardiac imaging, two 99mTc-labeled are tetrofosmin and sestamibi which are employed to ascertain the degree to which myocardial infarction is severe and also help to point out the regions of cardiac ischemia. Images are collected at the state of rest and after stressed activity of cardiac cells. This injection are administered when patient must have consumed any kind of fatty meal. This helps in hepatobiliary clearance of administered radiopharmaceuticals thus aid in getting better image. But it should not be administered when patients has consumed some drugs such as nitrates or calcium channel blockers.

1.2.5 Lungs

In case of lungs scan it is used for the purpose of diagnosis of any kind of embolism in pulmonary tract. Lung scan be of two types perfusion scan or ventilation scan. First, one 99mTc-labeled macroaggregated albumin is injected in the peripheral vein, which is then carried to the pulmonary artery system. It does not get absorbed rather it gets distributed evenly in the capillary bed and helps in diagnosis. Where blood flow is good there will be larger number of particles giving out radiation, whereas where there will less perfusion then less particles will be seen.

In case of ventilation scan, patient is made to inhale radioactive substance such as krypton or 99mTc-labeled DTPA aerosol. Image is obtained where air is seen circulating in lungs [5].

1.3 Adverse reactions

The most common adverse reaction associated with radiopharmaceuticals is sweating, nausea, dry mouth and rashes.

2. Recent approaches of injectable radiopharmaceuticals as nuclear medicine for imaging and therapy

The aim of this chapter is to explain about advancements the injectable of biomaterials or radiopharmaceuticals origin used in molecular imaging, therapy and clinical diagnosis. On the basis of intrinsic radiation form, radioisotopes can be divided into following type namely gamma (γ) ray emitters, beta (positron β+ or electron β−) particles emitters and alpha (α) particles emitters or their combinations. In clinical practice and pre-clinical animal studies, mostly used radionuclides are gamma ray emitters like Technetium-99m (99mTc), Iodine-123 (123I) and Galium-67 (67Ga), Positron-emitting radionuclides namely Fluorine-18 (18F), Oxygen-15 (15O), Carbon-11 (11C) and Zirconium 89 (89Zr). Some β-emitters are Rhenium-186/Rhenium-188 (186Re/188Re), Strontium-89 (89Sr), and Yttrium-90 (90Y). Examples of therapeutic α-emitters are Actinium-225 (225Ac), Bismuth-213 (213Bi) and Astatine-211 (211At) [6]. The injected radiopharmaceuticals can be in simple ionic form or in carrier complex form. Carrier complex has better targeting ability for certain tissues and cells and pathways of disease. These are some radioisotopes used for imaging are as follows (**Table 1**):

Organ	Isotope used/activity
Brain	In-113m/7–10 mCi
Kidney	Hg-197/150 mCi
Lungs	Tc-99/1 mCi I-131/0.15–0.3 mCi In-113/1 mCi
Spleen	Cr-51/0.3 mCi
Bone	Sr-85/0.1 mCi Sr-87/1 mCi F-18/1 mCi
Pancreas	Se-75/0.2 mCi
Placenta	Cr-51/0.05 mCi Tc-99/0.5–1 mCi

Table 1.
Radioisotope imaging [7].

In case of imaging, the major focus was development of 11C, 18F or 68Ga radiopharmaceuticals to be used in positron emission tomography (PET) and 99mTc-labeled agents for the used in single-photon emission computed tomography (SPECT) [8]. The merits associated with nuclear medicine are many such as it is noninvasive, it gives better in identifying exact region of tumor and beneficial for diagnosis of challenging diseases [9, 10]. In addition to this there is better quantitative analysis which is achieved with a numerous tools available. For example standard uptake values (SUVs) are taken in PET and in case of SPECT it is compared in vivo distribution of the injected materials [11]. There are some common nuclides mentioned in **Table 2** which are used in radiation therapy are:

Nuclide	Radiation	Half-Life	Treatment
32P	Β	14.3 d	Leukemia therapy
60Co	β, γ	5.3 yr	External cancer therapy
123I	Γ	13.3 yr	Thyroid therapy
131Cs	Γ	9.7 days	Prostate cancer therapy
192Ir	β, γ	74 d	Coronary disease

Table 2.
Radiation therapy [12].

This content focuses on the developments in field of imaging technology in relevance to imaging of radionuclide therapy.

2.1 SPECT and scintigraphy

This type of decay of radionuclides determines about the modality for imaging. Planar scintigraphy or SPECT is used for imaging of ^{177}Lu, ^{90}Y, and ^{131}I-which are used for radionuclide therapy. These emit γ-photons (or bremsstrahlung photons), which can be imaged by a γ-camera.

2.1.1 Current status

SPECT/CT systems which are used nowadays are used for both planar and tomographic imaging. Planar imaging is for acquiring whole-body images in when there is limitation of time. SPECT is meant for acquiring 3-dimensional data of structures which would otherwise overlap on each another on planar images.

Quantitative analysis of SPECT images is determined by converting the acquired counts in terms of distribution of absorbed dose (in Gy), which is beneficial for planning and dosimetry of therapy involving radionuclide. In clinical practice scatter correction is also implemented and is generally performed employing the triple-energy window method [13]. Quality of image can be enhanced by using resolution recovery. It is performed by characterizing the shape of the point-spread function accurately, that depends its distance from the camera and there is rotational variation due to the hexagonal pattern of the collimator septa. Reconstruction algorithm can be incorporated with point-spread function model subsequently [14].

Effects like scatter, blurring and attenuation which degrades image can be corrected to some extent, Although SPECT images can be degraded by partial-volume effects and quantification errors.

2.2 PET

^{18}F-FDG PET is used for many PET studies that are in the field of clinical practice and is employed for staging and follow-up post radionuclide therapy.

However, PET has application in planning of treatment, dosimetry, and assessment of treatment after radionuclide therapies.

2.2.1 Current status

Similar to SPECT quantitative PET is also used for correction techniques. Correction of attenuation for PET can be done through determination of the sonogram associated with attenuation correction, which works on the basis of co-registered CT data. Scatter correction is often done with single-scatter simulation method in clinical practice [15]. Correction for random counts is often done using delayed-event subtraction [16].

The difference in time between annihilation photons gives information regarding location of the annihilation and also about the line of response. Now time-of-flight information in the reconstruction at the time of back projection step enhances image quality. The availability of time-of-flight estimation has opened the opportunities for low positron abundance imaging isotopes like ^{90}Y.

As intrinsic resolution of PET detectors are not freely available, so shape of the point-spread function is used to improve the quality of images by incorporating it during reconstruction method. This is called as resolution recovery.

When there are high count rate radiation detection systems does not work properly due to dead-time effect caused by pulse pile-up. Because of these Dead-time losses are corrected regularly.

2.2.2 Advances

There are better quality of PET images with enhanced resolutions and sensitivity due to regular improvement in the instrument which provides precise determination of the SUV [17].

2.3 PET/MRI

The advantages of PET/MRI over PET/CT are higher soft-tissue contrast that is essential for planning of treatment, dosimetry, and assessment post radionuclide therapies. Additionally, for accurate dosimetry it is beneficial as it provides the simultaneous coregisteration of MR images. Also, MRI can be employed for determining the tolerable dose with least organ damaging activity of radionuclide. Along with it anatomic and molecular images acquisition provides better motion correction.

Integrating of PET and MRI modalities is challenging as there will be interference between both the modalities. For instance, photomultiplier tubes that are present in PET detectors malfunction in magnetic fields exerted by MRI. In addition to this, PET module affects the radiofrequency signal associated with MRI [18]. Due to this, the first generation of PET/MRI systems modalities were separated. Integration of PET detectors and MR scanner has been done to obtain PET and MR images simultaneously. Detector systems is avalanche photodiodes types or SiPMs types which are not sensitive to magnetic field. The simultaneous measurement provides better 4-dimensional acquisitions because of spatial agreement of PET and MRI data.

Disadvantages associated with PET/MRI are high costs and the ferromagnetic metallic implants which are used is contradictory to MRI. In addition to this it's challenging to correct attenuation of PET/MRI. For dosimetry it is essential to have accurate attenuation correction. As CT images are electron-density images and MR images are proton density image, CT image are better suited for attenuation

DOI: http://dx.doi.org/10.5772/intechopen.91868

correction. But MR images can be used for attenuation correction by using techniques such as segmentation-based or template- or atlas-based which derives electron density information from MR images [19]. Alternatively, estimation of the attenuation maps can be done by employing algorithms which uses the time-of-flight emission or transmission data [20].

2.4 Future perspectives

2.4.1 Simultaneous X-ray and nuclear imaging

Till today there are no real-time hybrid imaging modalities that can merge nuclear and anatomic for interventional purposes. Fluoroscopic imaging in combination with real-time nuclear imaging gives physicians with valuable information during procedures like as ^{90}Y liver radio embolization by image distribution of the radionuclide in association with the anatomy and the interventional instruments that enhances therapeutic efficiency. Image of same field can be seen by arranging X-ray tube, an X-ray detector, and a γ-camera in a single line [21].

3. Different types and applications of radioisotopes for imaging and therapy

S. no	Radioisotopes	Uses
1.	Calcium-47	Important aid to biomedical researchers studying cellular functions and bone formation in mammals
2.	Caesuim-137	Used to treat cancerous tumors and to measure correct dosages of radioactive pharmaceuticals
3.	Chromium-51	Used in research in red blood cells survival studies
4.	Cobalt-57	Used as a tracer to diagnose pernicious anemia
5.	Cobalt-60	Used to sterilize surgical instruments and used in cancer treatment, food irradiation and radiography
6.	Copper-67	When injected to monoclonal antibodies into a cancer patient, helps the antibodies bind to and destroy the tumor
7.	Gallium-67	Used in medical diagnosis
8.	Iodine-123	Widely used to diagnose thyroid disorders and other metabolic disorders including brain functions
9.	Iodine-125	Major diagnostic tool used in clinical test and to diagnose thyroid disorders. Also used in biomedical research
10.	Iodine-129	Used to check some radioactivity counters in in-vitro diagnostic testing laboratories
11.	Iodine-131	Used to treat thyroid disorders (Graves' disease)
12.	Iridium-192	In brachytherapy/tumor irradiation
13.	Phosphorous-32 and Phosphorous-33	Used in molecular biology and genetics research
14.	Technetium-99m	Most widely used radioactive pharmaceutical for diagnostic studies in nuclear medicine. Different chemical forms are used for brain, bone, liver, spleen and kidney imaging
15.	Uranium-234	Used in dental fixtures like crowns and dentures to provide a natural color and brightness
16.	Xenon-133	Used in nuclear medicine for lung ventilation and blood flow studies

3.1 Applications

Applications of different radioactive isotopes in nuclear medicine are [22]:

- Cobalt-60 is used in radiation therapy for prevention of cancer.
- Iodine-131 has been used for locating brain tumors, monitor activity of cardiac, liver and thyroid cells.
- Carbon-14 used for determining metabolic changes happening in patients of diabetes, gout and anemia.
- Carbon-11 is used to monitor organs during PET scan by tagging it into glucose.
- Thallium-201 has been in use for determining damage in heart tissue, detection of tumors.
- Technetium-99m act as radiotracer in medical diagnostics for obtaining the image of organs and study of blood flow. It also crucial for locating brain tumors and damaged heart cells [23].

4. Advantages and disadvantages of injectable radiopharmaceuticals

4.1 Properties of all radiopharmaceutical injectable

1. It should be sterile and free from Pyrogens. Sterility means absence of any living things even the spores or any related substances that can develop into something living. Culturing samples with special growth media is most common way to perform the assessment of sterility. Pyrogens are endotoxins that have the ability to cause pyrexia. They cannot be destroyed by autoclave and cannot be filtered. Testing for Pyrogens can be tested by using the rabbit test or the Limulus amebocyte lysate (LAL) test.

2. The isotonicity of injectable drug should be equal to 0.9% NaCl solution, and the pH should be 7.5.

3. In case of radioactive substance dose calibration should be done and it should be within ±10% of the prescribed dose. This calibration provides assurance that dose is as low as possible and it gives high quality image.

4.1.1 Advantages

- It is used for diagnosis and treatment of patients.
- It is commonly used to cure to cancers and can treat many other sites of disease.
- Treats tumor such as bone metastasis.
- Provide faster onset of relief from pain.
- Single dose is effective for some patients.
- Tests of nuclear medicine can be done on children.

- Nuclear medicine procedure less costly and painless.
- Nuclear medicine procedures are safe with no side effects [24].

4.1.2 Disadvantages

- Some allergic reactions can be seen.
- Risk of radiation is associated.
- Myelosuppression may occur before chemotherapy.
- Prolonged in convenience and discomfort can be experienced by patients due to administration of multiple fraction.
- Nuclear medicine tests cannot use for pregnant women because of potential risk to unborn babies.

5. Theranostics

Theranostics is a combination of two words **Thera**peutics and diag**nostics**. This is an emerging field of medicine where drugs and/or techniques are used in combination for treatment as well as treatment. It's a game changer as it provides diagnosis as well as therapy in single combination. It is economical as well as less time consuming. It uses PET scan to target tumor receptors which are present in tumor cell. If it is found in the cells radioactive drug is used to treat it. There are not much clinical trials found related to use of application of theranostics in prostate cancer by Australian Medicines Regulator—The Therapeutic Goods Administration (TGA) [25] (**Figure 2**).

5.1 Theranostics: Nuclear Medicine Imaging

The Nuclear Medicine Imaging approach is revolutionized by use theranostics [targeted therapeutic (Rx) + companion diagnostic (DX)] to establish tools for specific molecular targeting. It provides personalized treatment plan for the patient by targeting specific targets. Various department of nuclear science can utilize theranostic agents [26].

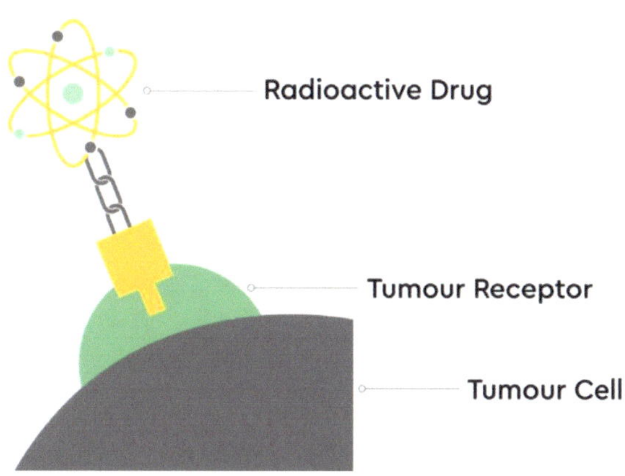

Figure 2.
Theranostics working on tumor cell.

5.2 Therapeutic bullets

Theranostics takes advantage of biological pathways specific to any system of human body to acquire diagnostic images. These images enhances the probability that the targeted therapeutic dosing of radiation that will only target disease part sparing the healthy one.

5.3 Nuclear Medicine Imaging

In past 100 years a similar kind of model for neuroendocrine tumors has been developed that has used radionuclide gallium-68. This PET radiotracer has been chelated to DOTA-octreotate and used for diagnosis of tumor with higher sensitivity compared to Indium-111 octreotide imaging.

The disease of patients can be determined by using the gallium-68 DOTA-TATE for targeting the somatostatin receptor volume and having image using hybrid scanner like PET-CT (Positron Emission Tomography-Computer Tomography). Lutetium Octreotate Therapy is a radiopharmaceuticals which emits beta radiation is available in 5 medical centers in north America and European medical centers [27].

Some of the milestones in the field of theranostics becoming personalized medicine are as follows:

- Lutetium PSMA therapy for metastatic or treatment-resistant prostate cancer
- Yttrium-90 SIRT therapy for liver cancer
- Iodine-131 therapy for thyrotoxicosis and thyroid cancer
- Radium-223 therapy for metastatic prostate cancer in bones
- Yttrium-90 radiosynovectomy therapy for inflammatory synovitis of joints

Theranostics targeted therapy is difficult in case of cancer treatment due to heterogeneity of cancer cells. Ibritumomab a monoclonal antibody detects B-cells and produces the beta/alpha-emitting radiometal for destroying the lymphoma. SPECT imaging confirms distribution of antibody in the body. The indium-111 combined with radionuclide yttrium-90 transports beta particles for killing the B-cells [28] (**Figure 3**).

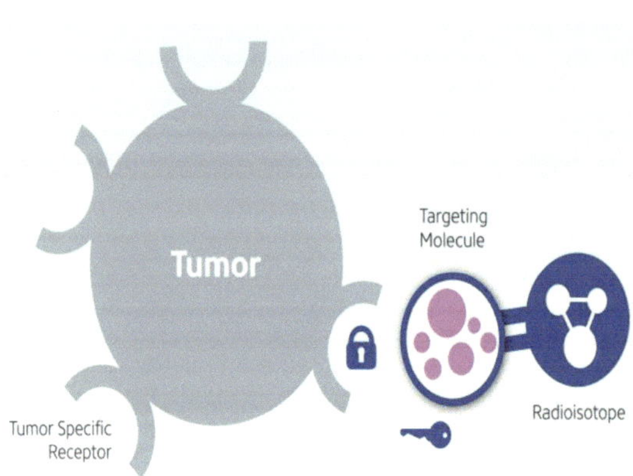

Figure 3.
Theranostics in cancer targeting and treatment.

5.4 Theranostics: Zevalin therapy

Zevalin therapy is used for determining the indications for relapsed or refractory, low-grade or follicular, B-cell non-Hodgkin's lymphoma. Zevalin is FDA approved for the treatment of relapsed or refractory low-grade follicular. In the year 2008 Zevalin was approved as the first-line drug for follicular lymphoma in the European Union.

5.4.1 Characteristics

5.4.1.1 Diagnostic component

The diagnostic component contains radiotracer, a contrast agent molecule, and a particulate system with either inherent physical property like optical, magnetic property or an acquired physical property such as, contrast enhanced ultrasound property or combinations of both. Combination systems exhibits dual functions like oximetry and detection in cellular and molecular imaging [29].

5.4.1.2 Therapeutic component

The therapeutic component includes drug molecule that is associated with diagnostic component or carrier system. Examples of the former are radiotracer-labeled non-peptide like gallium-68-labeled bisphosphonates for osteoblastic bone metastases and peptide-based molecules such as gallium-68-labeled somatostatin analogs for somatostatin receptor which targets neuroendocrine tumors. Examples of therapeutic components associated with a carrier system are where integrated entities are attaches to macromolecular carrier covalently. In addition to this, drug molecules co-encapsulation is done with diagnostic components such as chelated radiotracers and gadolinium (III), quantum dots, gold nanoparticle into particulate carrier systems namely polymeric nanospheres, liposomes, polymersomes, and mesoporous silica nanoparticles.

5.5 The application of theranostics in cancer

Cancer is a serious condition of heterogeneous group of diseases where there is uncontrolled and rapid cell growth. This is because of changes at genetic and/or epigenetic level in patient's body. Current treatment for cancer is chemotherapy, radiotherapy, immunotherapy and surgery.

Chemotherapy is not that much useful as a very low level of concentration of drug reaches the tumor. Moreover there is chances development of resistance during treatment and associated side effects. For example, chemotherapeutic agents known as taxanes have emerged as one of the most powerful classes of compounds to combat cancer, exhibiting a wide range of activity. The tubulin/microtubule complex has been proven to be a clinically useful antitumor target. The examples of chemotherapeutics that act *via* perturbation of tubulin polymerization include paclitaxel (Taxol®), docetaxel (Taxotere®), vinblastine, and discodermolide. First, docetaxel is a semi-synthetic derivative of paclitaxel. Next, vinblastine, unlike the other three compounds that all stabilize microtubules, aggregates tubulin and leads to microtubule depolymerisation. Randomized clinical trials evaluating docetaxel and paclitaxel in a first-line treatment setting for metastatic breast, lung, ovarian, and digestive cancers, as well as in the adjuvant setting for breast cancer, have confirmed that taxanes are leading contributors to the armamentarium of cancer treatments. Paclitaxel is used as a first-line chemotherapy treatment for NSCLC, but patients' acquired resistance becomes a critical problem.

Here nanomedicine is better as it allows molecular targeting to get higher concentrations of drug molecules at targeted site. Studies have been to make sure that required amount of drug reaches the site actively or passively which ensures better therapeutic index.

Few examples of nanomedicine in this context are polymeric micelles, polymer-drug conjugates and liposomes. Whereas traditional small molecular drugs n get eliminated from bloodstream quickly but nanomedicine possess longer half-lives.

Furthermore there is enhanced bioavailability and augmented tumor delivery. In addition to it integration of imaging and nanomedicine helps as diagnostic arm of theranostics. The advantages of using such strategy are immense, that will assist in management of oncogenic conditions with the help of theranostics [30].

Applications of theranostics in medicine include:

- It is a noninvasive molecular imaging method to evaluate of disease heterogeneity.
- Gives better idea about biodistribution and about accumulation of drug at target-site.
- Better understanding of process of local drug release.
- Facilitation of drug release (through application of stimuli-responsive theranostics).
- Prediction of drug responses and associated adverse effects with personalized therapies [31].

6. Health and safety

Radiopharmaceuticals are as safe as other medicine and before use they are tested carefully.

- The quantity of the pharmaceutical part of the radiopharmaceutical is very small, generally 1/10th of a millionth of an ounce. The risk of a reaction is 2–3 incidents per 100,000 injections, over 50% of which are rashes as compared to 2000–3000 per 100,000 injections of X-ray contrast media.
- For childrens most radiopharmaceuticals, the amount of radiation used for a diagnostic test is very low and considered safe [32].
- Radiopharmaceuticals usually are not recommended for use during pregnancy. This is to avoid exposing the fetus to radiation. His is specially important with radiopharmaceuticals that contain radioactive iodine, which can go to the baby's thyroid gland and in high enough amounts may cause thyroid damage.
- Although exposure to the radioactivity in very large doses can be harmful the radioactivity in radiopharmaceuticals is carefully selected by the nuclear medicine physician to be safe.
- If anybody will be receiving albumin in the form of radioiodinated albumin, technetium Tc 99m albumin aggregated, technetium Tc 99m albumin colloid,

or technetium Tc 99m albumin for test, Consult doctor if have ever had any unusual or allergic reaction to products containing human serum albumin [33].

- Side effects: when radiopharmaceuticals are used in very small doses to study an organ of the body, side effects are rare and usually involve an allergic reaction. These effects may occur almost immediately or a few minutes after the radiopharmaceutical is given.

7. Conclusion

In recent past radiopharmaceuticals made steady progress towards nuclear imaging and therapy. The benefit of molecular imaging and therapy can obtain when required amount of diagnostic probes reaches the targeted site. Effort have been taken in enhancing specificity of targeted radiotracers in both pre-clinical research and clinical trials. In recent discussions the advancement in the said field has been discussed taking into account multi-modal molecular imaging probes for sentinel lymph node mapping and image-guided surgery, radiotracers for targeted imaging of cancer and neurodegenerative diseases, along with probes for monitoring therapy responses. For better diagnosis and therapy design of radiopharmaceuticals as well as route of administration plays a major role. At last dose of radioactive medicine should be set with caution to prevent over exposure of patient, the principle of 'As Low as Reasonably Achievable' (ALARA) used for protection of employee as well as general public. The knowledge about medical physics is essential because of interactions between ionizing radiation and biological tissues. According to author we can be optimistic for the future growth of radiopharmaceuticals. This trend can be seen in recent future with the help of thriving research and fast translations into clinic. The high cost, demanding hardware requirements and specialized personnel training are major factors that may confine the development of radiopharmaceuticals. However, the huge needs for nuclear medicine from the public and the benefits to patient care far outweigh the risks.

Author details

Chanchal Deep Kaur[1*], Koushlesh Kumar Mishra[1], Anil Sahu[2], Rajnikant Panik[2], Pankaj Kashyap[2], Saraswati Prasad Mishra[3] and Anand Kumar[4]

1 Shri Rawatpura Sarkar Institute of Pharmacy, Kumhari, Chhattisgarh, India

2 Royal College of Pharmacy, Raipur, Chhattisgarh, India

3 RITEE Institute of Pharmacy, Raipur, Chhattisgarh, India

4 Sant Gahira Guru Vishwavidyalaya, Sarguja Ambikapur, Chhattisgarh, India

*Address all correspondence to: chanchaldeep@gmail.com

IntechOpen

© 2020 The Author(s). Licensee IntechOpen. This chapter is distributed under the terms of the Creative Commons Attribution License (http://creativecommons.org/licenses/by/3.0), which permits unrestricted use, distribution, and reproduction in any medium, provided the original work is properly cited. cc BY

References

[1] The Medicines Act 1968 (Application to Radiopharmaceutical-associated Products) Regulations. London: HMSO; 1992. Available from: www.legislation.gov.uk/uksi/1992/605/contents/made [Accessed: 03 June 2011]

[2] Theobald T. Sampson's Textbook of Radiopharmacy. 4th ed. London: Pharmaceutical Press; 2011

[3] Administration of Radioactive Substances Advisory Committee. Notes for Guidance on the Clinical Administration of Radiopharmaceuticals and Use of Sealed Radioactive Sources. 2006. Available from: www.arsac.org.uk/notes_for_guidance [Accessed: 03 June 2011]

[4] International Commission on Radiological Protection. Radiation dose to the patient from radiopharmaceuticals. Annals of the ICRP. 1988;**18**:1-4

[5] Chowdhury FU, Scarsbrook AF. The role of hybrid SPECT-CT in oncology: Current and emerging clinical applications. Clinical Radiology. 2008;**63**(3):241-251

[6] Hamoudeh M, Kamleh MA, Diab R, Fessi H. Advanced Drug Delivery Reviews. 2008;**60**(12): 1329-1346

[7] Sugashwaran J. Radioactivity—Natural and Artificial Radioactive Isotopes—Properties and Clinical Uses. Bangalore: Department of Radiation Oncology; 2014

[8] Holland JP, Williamson MJ, Lewis JS. Molecular Imaging. 2010;**9**(1):1-20

[9] Hoh CK, Schiepers C, Seltzer MA, Gambhir SS, Silverman DHS, Czernin J, et al. Seminars in Nuclear Medicine. 1997;**27**(2):94-106

[10] Öberg K, Eriksson B. Best Practice & Research Clinical Endocrinology & Metabolism. 2005;**19**(2):265-276

[11] Kinahan PE, Fletcher JW. Seminars in Ultrasound, CT and MRI. 2010;**31**(6): 496-505

[12] Sathekge M. Targeted radionuclide therapy has the potential to selectively deliver radiation to diseased cells with minimal toxicity to surrounding tissues. Continuing Medical Education. 2013;**31**(8)

[13] Ogawa K, Harata Y, Ichihara T, Kubo A, Hashimoto S. A practical method for position-dependent Compton-scatter correction in single photon emission CT. IEEE Transactions on Medical Imaging. 1991;**10**:408-412

[14] Zeng GL, Gullberg GT, Tsui BMW, Terry JA. Three-dimensional iterative reconstruction algorithms with attenuation and geometric point response correction. IEEE Transactions on Nuclear Science. 1991;**38**:693-702

[15] Zaidi H, Montandon M-L. Scatter compensation techniques in PET. PET Clinics. 2007;**2**:219-234

[16] Casey ME, Hoffman EJ. Quantitation in positron emission computed tomography: 7. A technique to reduce noise in accidental coincidence measurements and coincidence efficiency calibration. Journal of Computer Assisted Tomography. 1986;**10**:845-850

[17] Bockisch A, Freudenberg LS, Schmidt D, et al. Hybrid imaging by SPECT/CT and PET/CT: Proven outcomes in cancer imaging. Seminars in Nuclear Medicine. 2009;**39**(4):276-289

[18] Torigian DA, Zaidi H, Kwee TC, et al. PET/MR imaging: Technical

aspects and potential clinical applications. Radiology. 2013;**267**:26-44

[19] Keereman V, Mollet P, Berker Y, Schulz V, Vandenberghe S. Challenges and current methods for attenuation correction in PET/MR. Magma. 2013;**26**:81-98

[20] Nuyts J, Dupont P, Stroobants S, Benninck R, Mortelmans L, Suetens P. Simultaneous maximum a posteriori reconstruction of attenuation and activity distributions from emission sinograms. IEEE Transactions on Medical Imaging. 1999;**18**:393-403

[21] Beijst C, Elschot M, Viergever MA, de Jong HWAM. Toward simultaneous real-time fluoroscopic and nuclear imaging in the intervention room. Radiology. 2016;**278**:232-238

[22] Cuaron JJ, Hirsch JA, Medich DC, et al. A proposed methodology to select radioisotopes for use in radionuclide therapy. AJNR. American Journal of Neuroradiology. 2009;**30**:1824-1829

[23] Bhattacharyya S, Dixit M. Metallic radionuclides in the development of diagnostic and therapeutic radiopharmaceuticals. Dalton Transactions. 2011;**40**(23):6112-6128

[24] McCready VR. Milestones in nuclear medicine. European Journal of Nuclear Medicine. 2000;**27**(Suppl):S49-S79

[25] Baum RP, Kulkarni HR. Theranostics: From molecular imaging using Ga-68 labeled tracers and PET/CT to personalized radionuclide therapy—The Bad Berka experience. Theranostics. 2012;**2**:437-447

[26] Janib SM, Moses AS, MacKay JA. Imaging and drug delivery using theranostic nanoparticles. Advanced Drug Delivery Reviews. 2010;**62**:1052-1063

[27] Jokerst JV, Gambhir SS. Molecular imaging with theranostic nanoparticles. Accounts of Chemical Research. 2011;**44**:1050-1060

[28] Aerts A, Impens NR, Gijs M, et al. Biological carrier molecules of radiopharmaceuticals for molecular cancer imaging and targeted cancer therapy. Current Pharmaceutical Design. 2014;**20**(32):5218-5244

[29] Ma X, Zhao Y, Liang X-J. Theranostic nanoparticles engineered for clinic and pharmaceutics. Accounts of Chemical Research. 2011;**44**:1114-1122

[30] Moghimi SM, Hunter AC, Murray JC. Nanomedicine: Current status and future prospects. The FASEB Journal. 2005;**19**:311-330

[31] Leeds NE. The clinical application of radiopharmaceuticals. Drugs. 1990;**40**(5):713-721

[32] Volkert WA, Hoffman TJ. Therapeutic radiopharmaceuticals. Chemical Reviews. 1999;**99**:2269-2292

[33] Ercan MT, Caglar M. Therapeutic radiopharmaceuticals. Current Pharmaceutical Design. 2000;**6**: 1085-1121

Chapter 5

Localization Mechanisms of Radiopharmaceuticals

Sana Komal, Sana Nadeem, Zahra Faheem, Arouma Raza, Komal Sarwer, Hijab Umer, Samina Roohi and Syed Ali Raza Naqvi

Abstract

Scintigraphic techniques have opened a new era of developments in the localization of infectious and cancerous foci. Diseases area targeting mechanisms of radiopharmaceuticals encompasses visualization, characterization, and measurement of physiological and biological functioning at targeted sites in addition to measure the area and density of the disease. The accumulation of a radiopharmaceutical at specific organ is based upon numerous processes such as enzymatic interactions, receptor binding site, transport of chemical species and elimination of damaged cells from circulation by a normal metabolic process. PET and SPECT are developing scanning techniques that provides effective diagnostic tool to identify pathophysiology of diseased cells. In this chapter, we are exploring and explaining different mechanisms of radiopharmaceutical localization for imaging and therapeutic processes. The knowledge of these mechanisms will help to develop target based new radiopharmaceuticals using variety of medically used radioisotopes either for imaging or therapy of diseased cells.

Keywords: radiopharmaceuticals, SPECT imaging, antibiotics, infections, cancer

1. Introduction

Dysfunction and disruption of healthy physiological and biochemical cycles lead to the formation of malignancies. As the treatment of many diseases involves biochemical reactions so it may provide a basis for diagnosis. Several radiopharmaceuticals widely available that use to visualize the functioning and structure of body cells, tissues, and organs. These radiopharmaceuticals formulated for treating several malignancies, pain palliation due to bony metastases, joint diseases, and many other similar conditions. Nuclear medicine basically, a medical specialty comprises a carrier molecule and radiotracer that image the regional biochemistry of the body. The biochemical nature of carrier molecule and radiotracer; effects on organ uptake, retention, transportation and biodistribution towards targeted area. So, it's essential to know about the biochemistry of radiopharmaceuticals for better understanding [1]. Nuclear pharmacists must understand how radiopharmaceuticals localize and initiate its work, aka action mechanism. This expertise was required to assess the substrate specific and non-specific nature of labeled drug, its pharmacokinetics and biodistribution because life matters. As the radiopharmaceuticals provide us an opportunity for timely diagnostics using blood flow,

IntechOpen

multi-molecular cell localization, bio-energies, tissue metabolism, physiological functioning of the organ, intercellular and intracellular communicative pathways [2]. Different radiopharmaceuticals are used to image different organs based on the functioning of the organ. For example, the labeled iodine would be ideal for imaging thyroid malignancies, because inorganic iodine absorbed more in the thyroid. Similarly, radiolabeled phosphate widely used for the bone scan as it is observed that phosphate ions more accumulated in the bone. Hence one can use the same labeled atoms for organ imaging, which are more accumulated there.

A radiopharmaceuticals localization mechanism is specific to targeted organs depends on processes as varied as antigen–antibody reactions, physical particle trapping, receptor site binding, removal of deliberately damaged cells from circulation, and transportation of a chemical species across a cell membrane and into the cell via a normally operational metabolic cycle. Chemically, radiochemistry plays a crucial role in producing these compounds and in conducting quality assurance procedures to ensure purity [1, 3].

Some other factors also important for the selection and action of radiopharmaceuticals like for diagnosis gamma emitters were preferably choose (beta emitter in case of therapeutic), energy threshold 100–250 Kev, high T/NT ratio last but not least t_{eff} must be moderately long.

Furthermore, insoluble radiopharmaceuticals such as ^{99m}Tc-MAA and ^{99m}Tc-SC are used to represent the lungs and liver/spleen, diagnostic tests, respectively. Since it is well known that these two organs extract particles from the bloodstream, selection based entirely on particle size instead to chemical composition.

The mechanisms explained are not specific to radiopharmaceuticals, but these may be appropriate for some instances to explain the localization mechanisms of nuclear medicines. Radiopharmaceuticals are not limited to a mechanism but requires a combination of more than one mechanism. Lastly, a comprehensive overview of radiopharmaceuticals characteristics, their mode of action and detailed examples are given.

2. Mechanism of localization

The success of the molecular imaging technique using radioisotope labeled molecules commonly termed as radiopharmaceuticals relies on the mechanism of localization at disease cells. In the following sections we are explaining different mechanisms of radiopharmaceutical localization undertaken either for imaging process or therapy of diseases.

2.1 Compartmental localization

Generally, the phenomenon in which the desired species are disseminated in a bounded space is named as compartmentalization or may also be termed as compartmental localization and basically this bounded space is called as a compartment. Specifically, in radio pharmacy compartment-localization means to put a radiotracer in a bounded space and sustaining the tracer for time being enough to scan that bounded space. The bounded space contains fluids (either liquid or gas). The fluids of compartment move systematically in normal circumstances but the pathophysiological changes cause anomalies in the motion of compartmental fluids. These conditions if left unattended and untreated may become fatal. But the conventional diagnostic techniques fail to localize the exact location of abnormality, so, here radio pharmacy provides refuge and we can get exact pinpoint location along with treatment from molecular imaging.

The compartments in biological systems are: Vascular system (blood vessels), Airways of lungs, cerebrospinal fluid (CSF) space, Abdominal (peritoneal) cavity, Alimentary (digestive/GI) tract, urinary system, lymphatic vessels.

The compartmental localization could be in the form of:

a. Uniform distribution inside compartment

b. Non-uniform distribution within compartment

c. Outflow from compartment

d. Flow within the compartment

2.1.1 Uniform distribution inside compartment

Vascular system is the most typical example of uniform dispersion inside compartment. By utilizing the tracer dilution method blood volume could be analyzed quantitatively. A radiopharmaceutical named I-125 RISA (Radio-Iodinated Serum Albumin) diffuses uniformly in blood plasma, is employed to determine volume of plasma in blood.

- Cr-51 labeled RBCs is another radiotracer that is applied to evaluate the mass of red cells (volume of red cells in blood). This radiotracer distributes itself inside the blood's cellular part uniformly.

- Another radiotracer technetium-99 m labeled RBCs homogenously diffuses in blood, is used to evaluate expulsion fraction of left ventricle and movement of left ventricular wall by using gated blood-pool scanning.

2.1.2 Non-uniform distribution within compartment

Radiopharmaceuticals are not distributed equally every time. In some conditions they exhibit non-uniform dispersion, therefore showing disordered physiological process (due to some disease or injury). The increased concentration of a radiopharmaceutical in any organ or tissue corresponds to the disturbance in normal physiological function of that organ or tissue (pathologic changes).

Examples:

- Hemangioma is a condition in which a bright-red bump having extra blood vessels appears on skin and is quite rubbery. Extra blood vessels mean extra blood in that region. So, technetium-99 m labeled RBCs shows amplified localization in this region due to escalated volume of blood.

- Hydronephrosis is the inflammation of a kidney triggered by the accumulation of urine in kidney. This condition prevails when urine could not be drained out from kidney to bladder owing to some sort of obstruction or blockade. MAG3 and DTPA radiolabeled with ^{99m}Tc are used for its imaging. But, MAG3 has preference over DTPA due to its good output. Mercaptoacetyltriglycine (MAG3) is a peptide radiolabeled with ^{99m}Tc and it is released in kidney tubules. So, this increased volume of urine results in escalated amount of ^{99m}Tc-mertiatide (MAG3) or ^{99m}Tc-pentetate (DTPA) tracer in affected kidney.

The decreased concentration of the radiotracer in a compartmental cavity is usually the outcome of block in the cavity as mentioned in following examples:

- Xenon-133 ventilation imaging of lungs is used to confirm the obstruction in airways of lungs. This radiotracer will not be present past the block in the case of complete obstruction. While in partial hindrance, Xenon-133 would not be present in affected region after preliminary breathing but with time thru equilibrium rebreathing the radiotracer travel through the areas of partial hindrance.

- The obstruction in cerebrospinal fluid space could be monitored by intrathecal injecting ^{111}Indium-pentetate (DTPA). After injection ^{111}Indium-DTPA normally drifts up the spine and all over the brain. But in case of obstructing hydrocephalus, hindrance impedes the movement of ^{111}In-DTPA [4].

2.1.3 Outflow from the compartment

An uncharacteristic escape of content from compartmental space occurs owing to some pathologic changes (disturbances in normal physiological function). Radio pharmacy has a good lot of tracers that can precisely sense and find the location of compartmental leakage.

2.1.3.1 Mechanism of technetium-99 m labeled RBCs

Technetium-99 m labeled RBCs are used to foresee the exact location of Gastrointestinal bleeding. Because the blood from hemorrhaged vessel leaks-out and piles in GI-tract. So, radio-images using technetium-99 m labeled RBCs tracer shows the exact pinpoint location of hemorrhage.

After administration, technetium-99 m labeled RBCs speedily disperse in the vascular spaces. Small amount to activity could be observed in the urinary tract, that is due to free activity. No considerable GI bleeding is visualized in the early angiographs. But with time lapse the angiographs shows the bleeding in case of hemorrhage (blood move out of the disrupted area and the tracers in blood give exact scan of image [5].

The other examples include:

- ^{111}In-DTPA imaging is employed to demonstrate the leakage of cerebrospinal fluid.

- Post cholecystectomy, ^{99m}Tc-disofenin or ^{99m}Tc-mebrofenin could be used to monitor whether the bile is leaking out in abdomen or not.

- The ^{99m}Tc-MAG3, a peptide, binds ^{99m}Tc and could be employed to assess reno-vascular hypertension, kidney-transplant, hydronephrosis and urological anomalies. ^{99m}Tc-MAG3 (mercaptoacetyltriglycine) is also used to track leakage of urine into the abdominal cavity. Usually after kidney or urinary tract surgeries this complication occurs and urine seeps into the abdominal cavity.

2.1.4 Flow within the compartment

The changes in extent, rate and direction of compartmental flow is the consequence of some pathophysiological changes, that needs to be assessed and treated.

^{99m}Tc-sulfur colloids is preferably used for studying the rate at which gastric contents are emptied in the stomach by. The reason why ^{99m}Tc-sulfur colloid is suited for this study is that it is not absorbed by Gastrointestinal tract. For assessment of solid emptying rate ^{99m}Tc-sulfur colloid is bound in scrambled eggs, while for liquid emptying rate ^{99m}Tc-sulfur colloid is mixed in drinking water. Then experimental values are compared to normal values with a margin of ±2 standard deviation. The presence and rate of back reflux of contents (due to infections) of urinary bladder to kidney is also studied by the scans taken at specific time lapse using ^{99m}Tc-sulfur colloid (SC). This tracer is implanted by means of a catheter in bladder [6].

2.2 Passive diffusion/simple diffusion

Passive diffusion refers to the random motion from higher to lower concentration of molecules to attain uniformity. Diffusion of tea into water from teabag is most common example of passive diffusion. But typically, in a biologic system this movement comprises motion of molecules across the membrane. Factors like pH, ionization, size of molecule and lipid solubility affect the mobility of molecules to move across the membranes.

Lipid solubility is the primary factor as phospholipids, glycolipids, sphingolipids, and sterols are the common types of lipids that make up membranes, of which phospholipid is the chief constituent. So, only the molecules that are soluble in lipids (lipophilic) could move across the membranes while polar hydrophilic molecules could not cross the membrane system.

pH and ionization impact also influence the mobility of molecules, as all molecules bear different charge (either neutral or charged according to pH). As pH varies the ionization state also varies. Like amines maybe neutral at high pH values and protonates at low pH values. So, according to the pH of surrounding, molecule could not move across membrane when ionized state (hydrophilic), but same molecule could pass when in non-ionizes state (lipophilic).

Size of molecules is another important parameter, allowing only molecules of certain size to pass through the pores on membranous surface. Generally, the particles that weigh less than 80 Daltons could pass only, the entry of molecules greater than this size is thus restricted.

There are certain characteristics of passive diffusion:

- Concentration gradient is required for this type of movement. The membranes in human body segregates this concentration gradient so, in biologic systems it is movement across the membrane (from higher to lower concentration).
- It is fast at high conc. Gradient and slow at low conc. Gradient.
- It does not need any sort of input as it is a passive method.
- It is a non-selective process because no carriers or receptors are included in this method.

Many radiotracers are localized in the targeted organs by mechanism of passive diffusion. And its flow is invariably from areas of high tracer concentration to lower. Initially, diffusion rate is in direct proportionality to the tracer concentration, until equilibrium is achieved. ^{133}Xe,^{127}Xe, and ^{81m}Kr are commonly used for ventilation and have non-reactive lipophilic nature. After administering the tracer via inhalation, diffusion process operates, and the ventilation gas is scattered in airways of lungs. The flow is smooth until and unless discontinued due to the presence of hinderance in airways. After entering the pulmonary circulation, gases leave lungs by alveolar-capillary diffusion method.

2.2.1 Mechanism of ^{99m}Tc-DTPA (diethylene triamine penta-acetic acid)

A chief factor that has a key role in localization mechanism of radio tracer in brain region is barrier of blood and brain (brain–blood barrier/BBB). It is basically a uniform film of endothelial cells belonging to cerebral vessels, restricting the diffusion of lipophobic molecules, and allowing only lipophilic ones. Due to some physiological abnormalities, this barrier is interrupted allowing the diffusion of hydrophilic molecules in tissues of brain. Oxygen, electrolytes, CO, glucose, water and other smaller molecules diffuses passively in across barrier and use active mechanism to move in the neural cells, while immuno-globulins (large particles), many lipophobic radiotracers and other lipophobic (hydrophilic) particles cannot cross the barrier under normal circumstances but in situations when barrier is disrupted the radiotracers accumulate at the area of tumor/abnormality easily, showing a + scan.

A typical radiopharmaceutical for brain imaging by ^{99m}Tc-DTPA. Normally, it cannot diffuse across barrier easily because of its lipophobic nature (See **Figure 1(A)**), but in abnormalities like tumor and infections the barrier is disturbed, so, ^{99m}Tc-DTPA move passively across barrier and amass in the infected area of brain (See **Figure 1(B)**). Its biologic half-life is 1–2 hours, halftime for clearance of plasma is 70 minutes and in 24 hours 90% of the tracer is eliminated by urinary system.

10–20 millicurie of ^{99m}Tc-DTPA is injected intra-venously in the body and after an hour scanned via gamma cameras. If the scan shows no agglomeration of radiotracer in brain, it means that the barrier is intact, and the tracer was not able to past across the barrier. But if the scans show tracer concentration in the cells of brain it means the barrier is no more intact and is prevailed by anomalies. So, the tracer highlights the affected areas as hot-spots [7].

Other examples:

Other radiotracers that are involved in such type of study (that localize passively in brain) are ^{99m}Tc-glucoheptonate (GH), ^{123}I-serum albumin, technetium pertechnetate ($^{99m}TcO_4^-$) [9], Thallous chloride Tl-201 [10, 11], Gallium citrate Ga-67 [12].

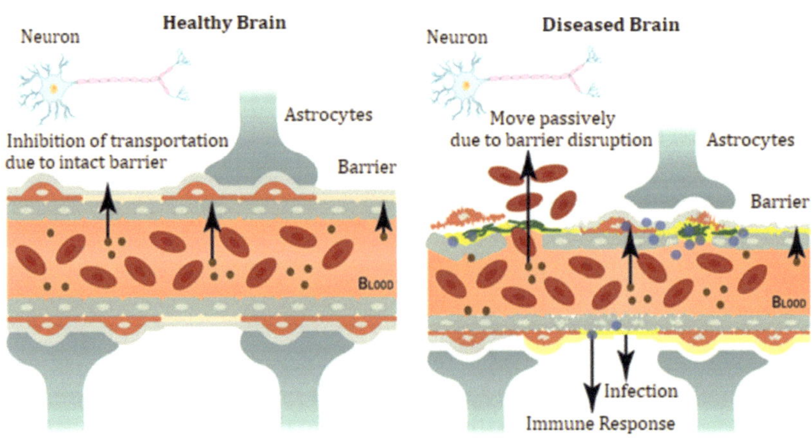

Figure 1.
(A) Illustration of intact barrier in the brain cells that do not allow ^{99m}Tc-DTPA to diffuse, (B) disruption of barrier in the brain cells [8].

2.2.2 Mechanism of ^{99m}Tc- Sestamibi

^{99m}Tc labeled cationic, lipophilic tracers like furifosmin, tetrofosmin and Sestamibi for myocardial perfusion imaging have been established. ^{99m}Tc-Sestamibi is some-what similar to cationic $^{201}Tl^{+}$ but Sestamibi transport across the membrane only involves passive diffusion [13]. In start, it was assumed that the uptake of technetium labeled Sestamibi by the myocardial cells is primarily because of binding of lipid constituents to the membrane of cell. This ambiguity was later cleared that uptake was not because of membrane's binding to lipid constituent, instead the cellular entry is chiefly linked to mitochondria and its negative potential of inner membrane. About 90% of uptake was linked to mitochondria [14] (See **Figure 2(A)**). It was studied that the upholding of technetium labeled Sestamibi is not specific to tumor of some organs, rather it is a general mechanism.

^{99m}Tc- Sestamibi moves passively from blood to tumor and amass in the cancers that have low multidrug-resistant pump expression and more mitochondria making cancers susceptible to precise diagnosis. But in most cases, the resistance pump dominates over mitochondrial presence making cancers non-susceptible to ^{99m}Tc-Sestamibi, because the resistance pumps eject the radiotracer out of the cell [15]. So, the upholding status of this radiotracer reflects the membrane permeability of mitochondria and the mitochondrial potentials. Alterations due to cancers leads to dys-functioning of mitochondria that consequently cause decreased uptake of tracer [16] (See **Figure 2(B)**). The decreased upholding of technetium Sestamibi in the terms of chemotherapy (after chemotherapeutic session) is correlated to the over-expression of multidrug-resistant proteins. So, the cancers which do not uphold this tracer are not prone to chemotherapy.

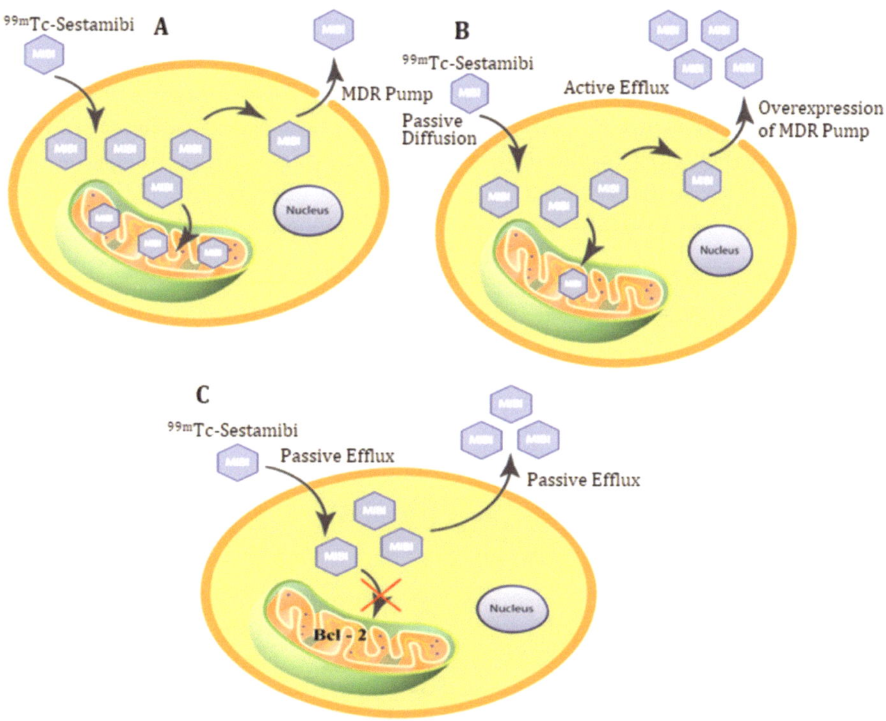

Figure 2.
(A) Normal binding of ^{99m}Tc- Sestamibi to mitochondria, (B) over-expression of resistance pump that quickly removes ^{99m}Tc-sestamibi out of cell, (C) effect of Bcl-2, an anti-apoptotic protein; that halts the binding of ^{99m}Tc-sestamibi to mitochondria [17].

The other possibility is that the protein that prevents the induction of apoptosis (Bcl-2, prevents the membrane permeability of mitochondria) maybe over expressed, halting the entry of radiotracers in mitochondria [18] (See **Figure 2(C)**).

Few compounds to suppress/neutralize the effects of anti-apoptotic protein have been subjected to clinical trials. The purpose for this is to monitor the credibility and efficacy of ongoing therapeutic procedure.

2.3 Phagocytosis

The word "Phagocytosis" derived from Greek language that translate as "CELL EATING" (a procedure in which cell engulfs a particle and internalizes it). A prime example involves Kupffer cells (that present in the lining of liver and involve in the breakdown of red blood cells also known as phagocytic cells) in the reticuloendothelial system entrapped the radio-labeled colloidal particles following an intravenous injection [19]. The particle size of radiolabeled colloidal suspensions is usually between 0.05 to 4 μm. ^{99m}Tc-macro-aggregated albumin and ^{99m}Tc-sulfur colloid are mostly used as phagocytic agents and their size ranging from approximately 0.1–2.0 μm are able to leave the circulation via the sinusoidal type capillary structures in the liver, spleen, and bone marrow [20]. There is inverse relation between particle size and its bone marrow uptake that is why the larger particles will localize in spleen and liver.

The diameter of capillary is about seven micro-meters which is larger than particle size, capillary blockade does not occur. Opsonin (serum specific protein) may interrelate and provide coating to the colloids so that may be recognize by receptors site; then, engulf and removed from circulation by cells of the reticuloendothelial system as shown in **Figure 3** [21].

Macrophages in liver sinusoids (Kupffer cells) and macrophages in spleen (reticular cells) accumulate the particles by phagocytosis. In a liver scan with ^{99m}Tc-sulfur colloid cold lesions identified may be due to intra hepatic tumor displacing normal distribution of reticuloendothelial system's cells. Similarly, decreased reticuloendothelial system functioning may appear as radiation damage in bone marrow and liver shown as cold areas in scan results. Patients having melanoma and breast cancer, ^{99m}Tc-SC has been widely used in lympho-scintigraphy for the identification of sentinel node which is the first lymph node to receive lymphatic drainage from tumor cells [22].

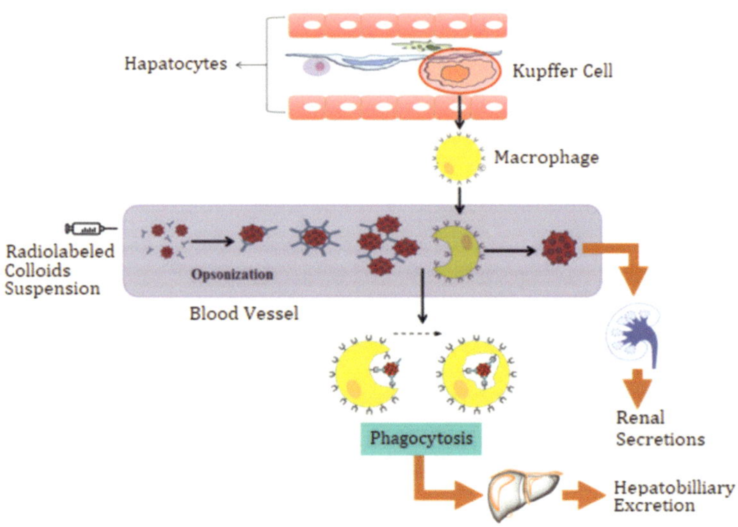

Figure 3.
Phagocytosis process through macrophages of liver (Kupffer cells) present in the lining of liver [20].

Distribution in the endothelial system is typically Five percent in marrow, Ten percent in spleen and eighty-five percent in liver. The t_{biol} of macro-aggregated albumin is 6–12 hours which is infinitely short as compared to t_{biol} of ^{99m}Tc-sulfur colloid in the liver. T ½ of clearance from the blood pool is 2.5 min; so, in approximately ten minutes only 6% remains in blood stream. Imaging must begin after 5–10 minutes of intravenous colloidal injection [23].

The radiopharmaceutical, Tc-99 m sulfur colloid, is localized by this mechanism used for liver scans. Cyst, tumor abscess or hemangioma are focal areas of lacking phagocytic cells will be demonstrated as "Areas of lack uptake". There will be a colloid shift if liver is poorly functioning such as with cirrhosis or hepatitis [22, 24].

2.4 Capillary blockade

This technique most precisely depends upon the phenomenon of micro-embolization (trapping the radiolabeled particles in the capillary bed) used to determine perfusion of organ such as brain, heart, and lung. For pulmonary perfusion studies commonly used radiolabeled particles is Technetium labeled macro aggregated albumin particles. ^{99m}Tc-MAA particles have diameter of about 10–50 μm while, pre-capillaries and capillaries have a mean diameter of 20–25 μm and 8 μm, respectively. Therefore, intravenous injection of ^{99m}Tc-MAA particles block the blood flow to the distal region of lung by physically trapped in arterio-capillary beds as shown in **Figure 4** [19, 25].

Smaller particles pass through the pulmonary capillaries and are extracted by the reticuloendothelial system in the body. Therefore, the mechanism of localization of particles in lungs is purely a mechanical process, called capillary blockade. In experimental animal studies, gold standard for determination of organ perfusion is radiolabeled microspheres with varying particle diameter and physical half-lives [27].

The first encountered capillary beds are the lungs when such sized particles injected intravenously. For perfusion lung scan radiolabeled particles (Tc-99 m

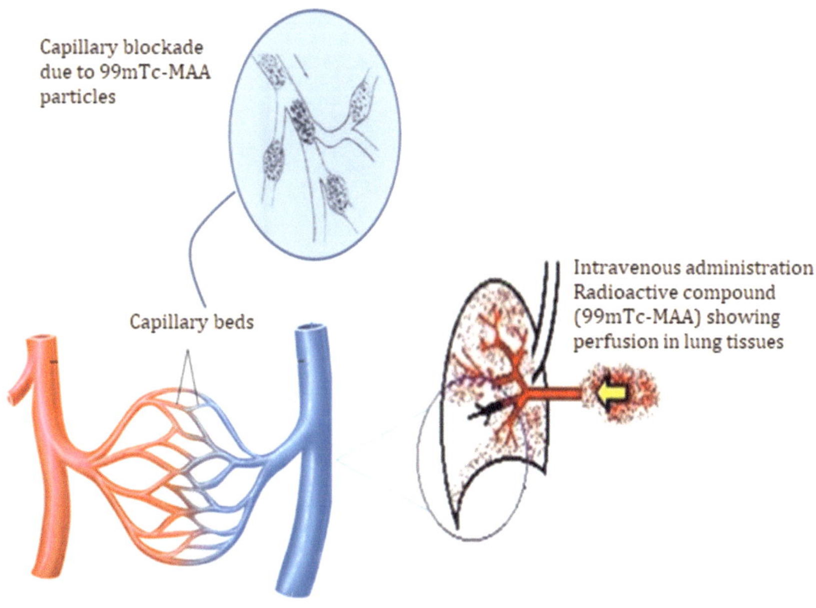

Figure 4.
Illustration of capillary blockade due to ^{99m}Tc-MAA accumulation in capillary beds [26].

macro-aggregated albumin) have been used. This delivery mechanism necessarily involves to the capillary beds via blood flow, localization of Tc-99 m MAA is a surrogate for relative blood flow in lungs. Therefore, this perfusion lung scan with Tc-99 m MAA aggregates also used to assess blood flow in pulmonary arteries. A similar procedure in which Tc-99 m MAA is injected in hepatic artery through a catheter, it is delivered via hepatic blood flow to the capillaries in the liver [19, 28].

2.5 Cell sequestration

Potentially saturable mechanism that is mostly associated with spleen and refers to the process where damaged and old RBC's removed from circulation [29]. It is unlikely for the relatively small numbers of cells used for imaging. The radiopharmaceutical preparation is carried out by in vitro labeling of red blood cells with technetium-99 m using modified Brookhaven labeling method and then damaging them by heating at 49°C for fifteen minutes (**Figure 5**).

2.6 Ion exchange

Ion exchange is a mechanism of localization in which ions exchange between a complex like hydroxyapatite and electrolyte solution. ^{18}F radioisotope is typically used for imaging metastatic and primary tumors present in bone. In ^{18}F-NaF the mechanism of localization followed by this radiopharmaceutical is Ion exchange mechanism and is used for studying metabolism of bones and also for bone imaging [19]. ^{18}F obtained from cyclotron is diluted by using 5 mL of sterile water and then passed through a sealed unit containing cation exchanger and then anion exchanger. To obtain ^{18}F-NaF, 10 ml saline (NaCl) is added in anion exchanger. And then eluted ^{18}F-NaF from anion exchanger is ready to inject in patients. The localization mechanism of ^{18}F-NaF in infected area involves the exchange of fluorine anion (F^-) from hydroxyl group (OH^-) in hydroxyapatite a bone crystal [Ca_{10} $(PO_4)_6$ $(OH)_2$]. After the exchange of F^- with OH^-, fluoroapatite [Ca_{10} $(PO_4)_6$ $(F)_2$] is formed as shown in **Figure 6** [1].

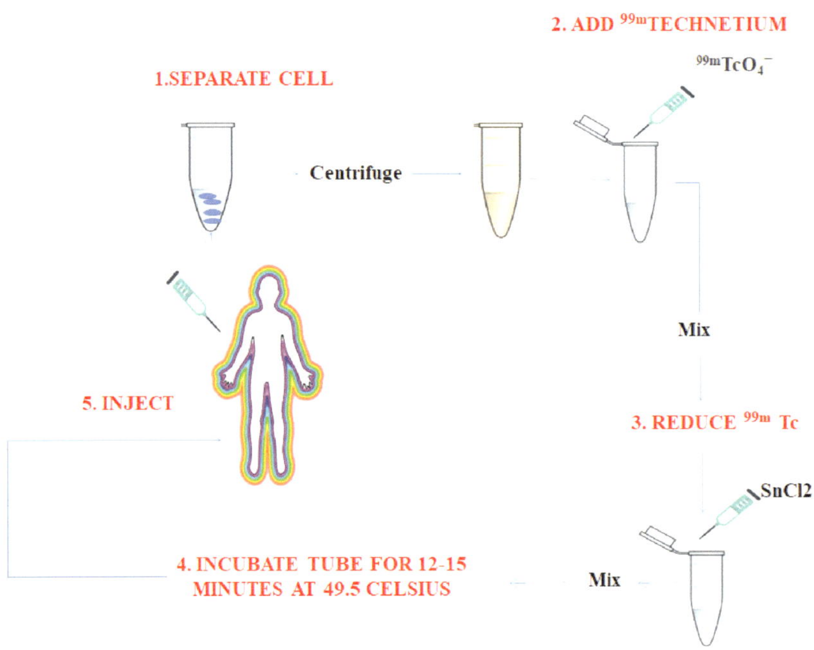

Figure 5.
Schematic explanation of ^{99m}Tc-DRBC preparation [30].

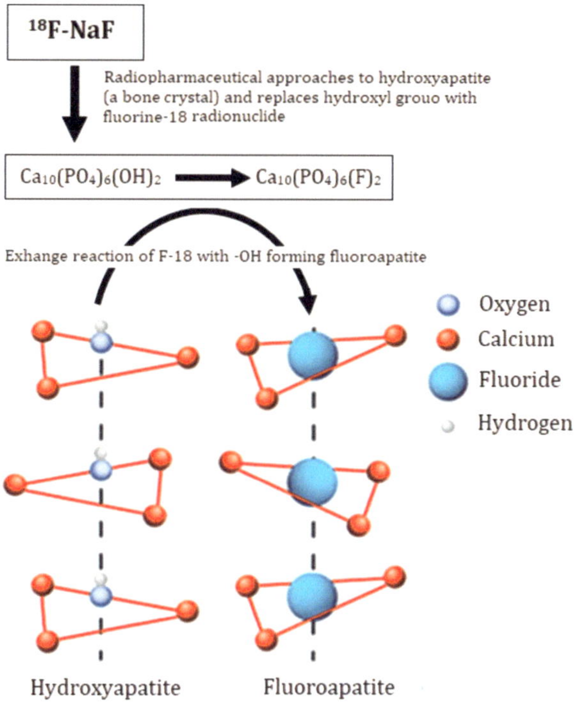

Figure 6.
Ion exchange mechanism of ^{18}F-NaF for bone deposition [31].

When ^{18}F-NaF injected in the body of patient its distribution depends on the blood flow of body and the amount of ^{18}F-NaF distributed in different bones at different ratio. In bone marrow the uptake of radioisotope is almost negligible. ^{18}F-NaF can easily diffuse through membrane and almost 30% radiotracer present in erythrocytes. ^{18}F-NaF has a fast plasma clearance rate. For bone deposition ^{18}F-NaF must pass through extracellular fluid with the help of plasma. The incorporation of fluoroapatite in bone in a slow process and it depends on the area of infected bone. In case of malignant bone disorder, the incorporation time of fluoroapatite is high. Fluoroapatite has low binding with plasma protein and rapidly clear from non-targeted area. After 40–45 minutes of radiotracer injection, fluoroapatite permits the whole body imaging [32].

2.7 Chemisorption

Chemisorption also known as physiochemical adsorption is localization mechanism refers to the binding of phosphate-type compounds like methylene diphosphate (MDP), pyrophosphate (PYP) and hydroxy diphosphate (HDP) onto the bone surface. So, with the increase in bone metabolism like tumor, fracture and infection, surface area increases and hence there is enhanced accumulation of radiopharmaceutical at that surface. ^{99m}Tc-MDP, ^{99m}Tc-PYP, and ^{99m}Tc-HDP all bind to tissues of bone by this mechanism [19].

The administration of radiopharmaceuticals with low-energy photons that are attached chemically to moiety having affinity with hydroxyapatite a bone mineral. This attachment permits selective radiation dose to the area of interest with no or minimum radiation dose to the non-infected tissues. Out of 100%, only 40–50% dose of injected radiopharmaceutical localizes in bone and the remaining 50–60% dose is excreted from body through kidneys. Since, the radiopharmaceutical uptake in bone is low, so imaging starts after three hours of post injection [33].

2.7.1 Chemisorption mechanism of ^{99m}Tc-PYP

^{99m}Tc-PYP is used for the acute myocardial infarction imaging is an example of Chemisorption mechanism of localization. Myocardial infarction starts when myocardial cells turn out to be necrotic, calcium ions influx create into the cells. Circulating phosphate ions present in body reacts with the Ca^{2+} ions and $Ca_3(PO_4)_2$ crystals are formed. Resulting calcium phosphate crystals formed hydroxyapatite present on bone tissues. ^{99m}Tc-PYP binds irreversibly and avidly to calcium phosphate crystals at the infarct periphery where some perfusion is maintained as shown in **Figure 7**. After two hours of post injection imaging takes place [34].

2.8 Filtration

Filtration is denoted as a significant case of diffusion in which carrier molecules are compelled to progress by an osmotic or hydrostatic pressure gradient through several channels and pores. The significant example of this process explained is by glomerular filtration of kidney. Radiopharmaceuticals are effectively employed in renal imaging and in the determination of renal morphology or renal functioning. Two physiological mechanisms such as glomerular filtration and tubular secretion are accountable for renal imaging. Agents cleared by glomerular filtration are further utilized in investigating the glomerular filtration rate (GFR) [19].

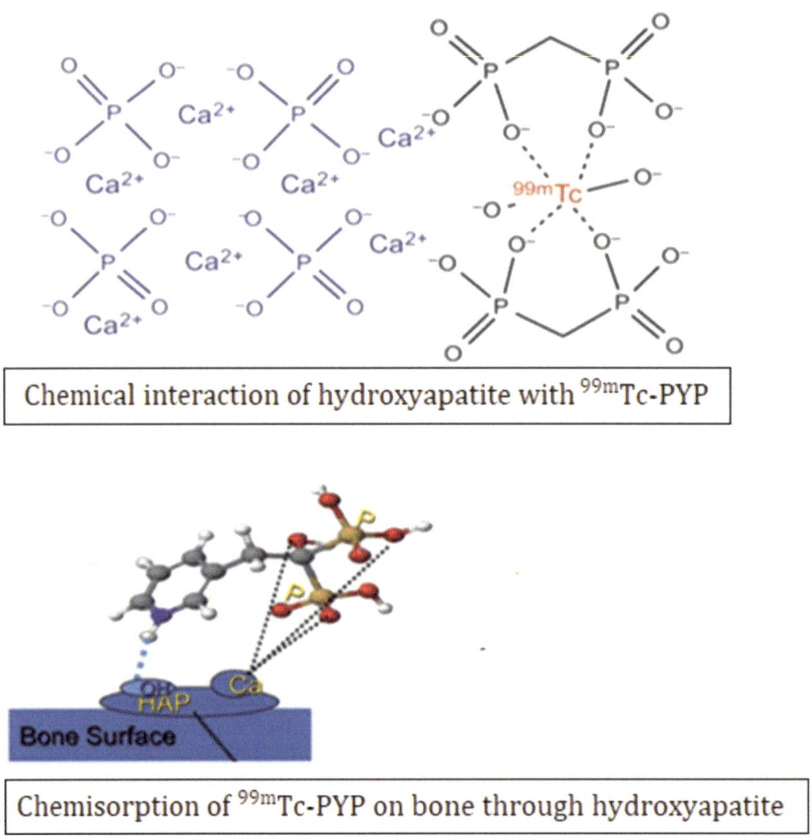

Figure 7.
Systematic representation of chemisorption of ^{99m}Tc-PYP [35].

There are two factors that are primarily concerned for the glomerular filtration of kidney comprising radiopharmaceuticals. First factor is the availability, only those molecules are liable for filtration that are freed in plasma and are not protein bounded. Second factor required for glomerular filtration is the pore size versus molecular size. Usually, only small hydrophilic molecules having a size less than 5000 are capable of disseminating through glomerular pores [36].

Some other factors are also involved in this glomerular filtration mechanism. Some pressure gradient or force is necessity for filtration while in the case of glomerular filtration, this specified force is provided by blood pressure however it does not demand any indigenous involvement of external output or energy. Moreover, filtration is non-selective due to the non-involvement of any receptors, transporters or carrier molecules [37].

Various radiopharmaceuticals are excreted partially by glomerular filtration, but the radiopharmaceutical most employed for renal imaging glomerular function is Tc-99 m DTPA. Renal DTPA can be determined from estimating the activity in multiple or single blood samples, the elimination of activity from tissue or blood and from the emergence of tracer particles in urine [19]. Example of Filtration process is depicted as shown in **Figure 8**.

Some other radiopharmaceuticals excreted indigenously during glomerular filtration are ^{99m}Tc- MAG3 and EC (ethylene di-cysteine) for tubular secretion, ^{131}I and ^{123}I for Tubular (80%) and glomerular (20%), ^{99m}Tc-DMSA for cortical binding (50%), and ^{99m}Tc-GHA for cortical binding (20%) and glomerular filtration (80%) as shown in **Figure 9**.

2.9 Active transport

Active transport is carrier mediated, metabolic, energy dependent pathway in a body to move forward a radiopharmaceutical across a cell membrane into a cell. The energy utilized during this reaction comes from ATP that allows the transport of molecules against a concentration gradient. It is carrier selective, which explicates fitting of small number of molecules into a specific carrier and makes it possible to accomplish saturation i.e. maximum response provided when all the carriers are engaged [19].

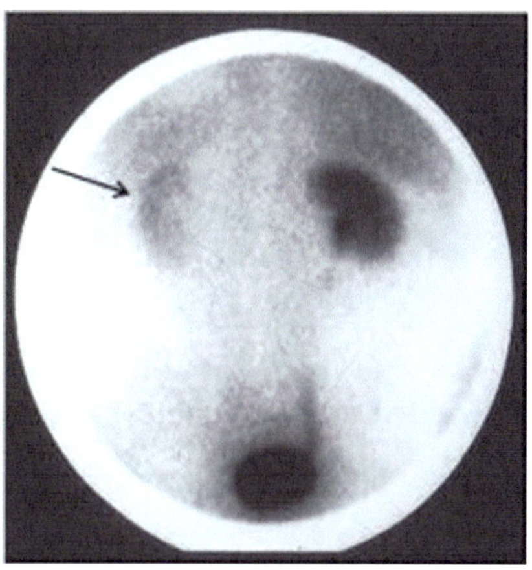

Figure 8.
Pre-treatment was done with captopril (an ACE inhibitor used for decreasing pressure on blood vessels), glomerular filtration of Tc-99 m DTPA is decreased as seen in the left kidney (arrow). Captopril employed, blocked the compensation mechanism triggered by left kidney ensuring a decreased pressure in the left kidney [19].

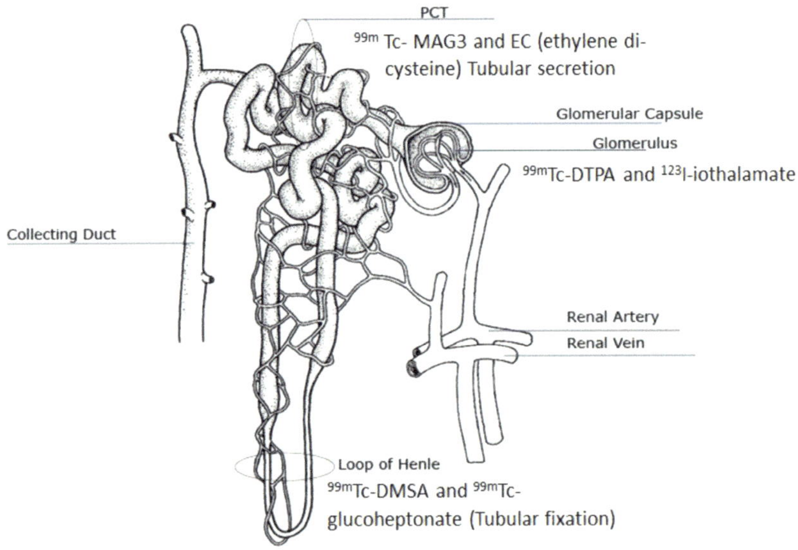

Figure 9.
Different mechanism of renal radiopharmaceutical excretion and uptake, including glomerular filtration, cortical binding and tubular secretion [38].

Concentration of iodide in the thyroid gland is an eminent example of active transport. Iodide ions are conveyed into thyroid cells by the Na^{+}/I^{-} symporter. Therefore, I-123 and I-131 (radioisotopes of iodine) are suitable radiopharmaceuticals to assess thyroid functioning [3]. Furthermore, Tc-99 m pertechnetate has almost same negative charge and ionic radius, hence it is too transported like iodide as shown in **Figure 10**.

It is highly significant that high concentrations of iodide (in the form of injections of iodinated contras media) in the blood, will competitively prevent thyroid uptake of these radiopharmaceuticals. Firstly, iodide is trapped producing an intermediate thyroglobulin and is eventually converted into T3 & T4. Preliminary, localized in thyroids, parotids and stomach and ultimately cleared through kidneys as shown in **Figure 10** [39].

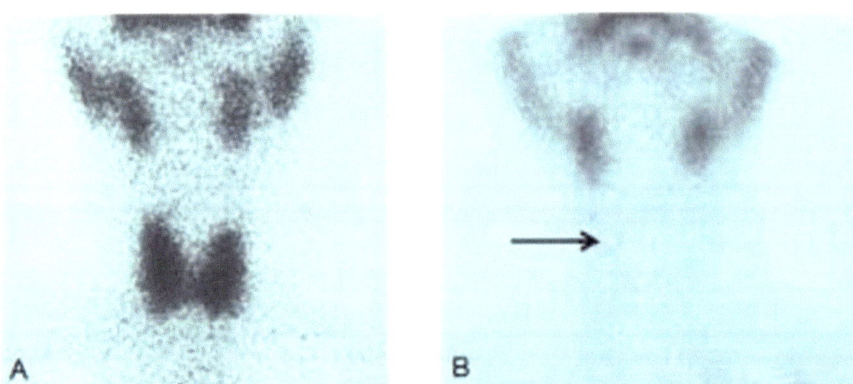

Figure 10.
(A) Regular uptake of Tc-99 m pertechnetate in thyroid (and salivary glands). (B) Absent uptake of thyroid (arrow) of Tc-99 m pertechnetate in an iodinated x-ray contrast media administered patient a few days earlier [19].

Glucose absorption from the GI tract into the blood and then reabsorption of glomerular-filtered glucose back into the blood by the distal renal tubules is another example of active transport. A sodium-dependent glucose cotransporter (SGLT) is employed to perform this function. Even though F-18 FDG is not voluntarily transported by SGLTs, glomerular filtered F-18 FDG residues in the urinary tract and flows to the bladder. Eventually, F-18 FDG do not perform the same function as glucose that is being reabsorbed into the blood [19] (**Figure 11**).

A third example of active transport is the Na+/K+ (sodium/potassium) pump, due to its significance in the heart muscle. Thallous chloride has extensively employed for myocardial perfusion scans. However, due to similar ionic size of thallous ion as potassium ion, it fits in place of potassium ion in sodium/potassium pump. Therefore, heart muscles reflect coronary perfusions.

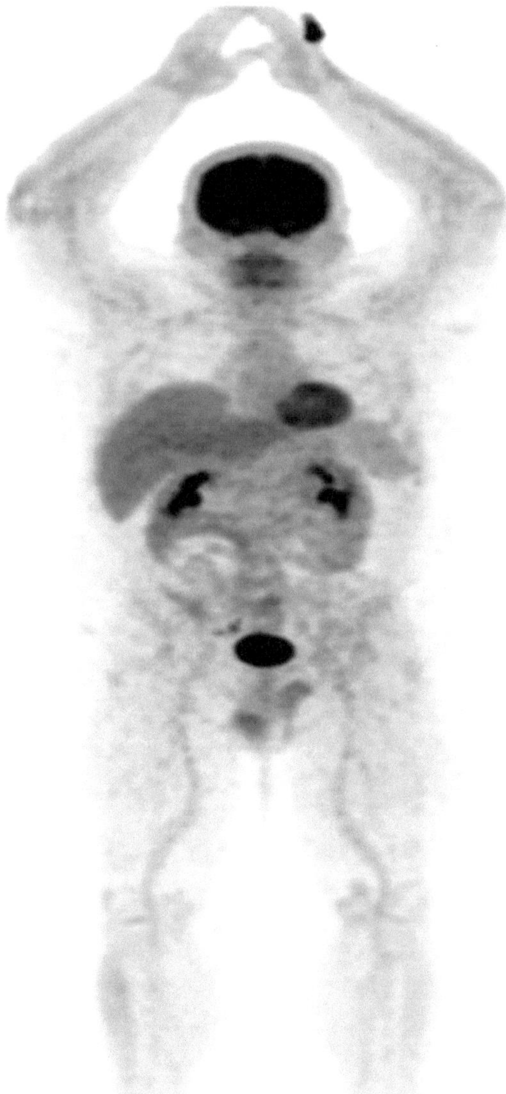

Figure 11.
Following injection of F-18 FDG in a normal patient, there is high uptake in brain, variable uptake in heart (high uptake in this patient), and moderate uptake in liver, GI tract, and marrow [19].

A second radiopharmaceutical is rubidium chloride which falls just below the potassium in periodic table has somewhat similar properties and fits in sodium/potassium pump, thus utilizing for PET myocardial perfusion scans [39].

2.10 Facilitated diffusion

A type of carrier-mediated transport across membranes is known as facilitated diffusion. Essentially, a carrier is utilized to carry the molecule across the membrane so, it is a selective carrier membrane (i.e., only certain molecules fit into the carrier). Consequently, it is inhibited by the presence of similar molecules that also fit into the carrier. Saturation can be achieved to maximum due to limited number of carriers. Facilitated diffusion expends passive so it entails a concentration gradient for its functioning. However, external energy is not employed in facilitated diffusion.

Glucose is the key example of facilitated diffusion. Glucose move into the cells by transmembrane protein transporters [GLUT]. Similarly, radiolabeled analog of glucose F-18 fludeoxyglucose (FDG), goes into the cells via the glucose transporters [GLUT]. After entering the cell, both glucose and FDG are phosphorylated by hexokinase. Glucose-6-phosphate then enters the glycolytic pathway. But the metabolism of FDG-6-phosphate is further blocked, so FDG is reserved in the cells. It is significant to summon up that glucose and FDG are competing for GLUT transporters, consequently prominent blood levels of glucose will reduce the cellular uptake of FDG [19] (See **Figure 12**).

2.11 Cellular migration

A physiological migration directed by cell especially in response to some stimuli. The principle example is taxis of WBCs in response to inflammatory chemokines and cytokines. Ex-vivo labeling of ^{99m}Tc-HMPAO and ^{111}In-oxyquinoline with phagocytic

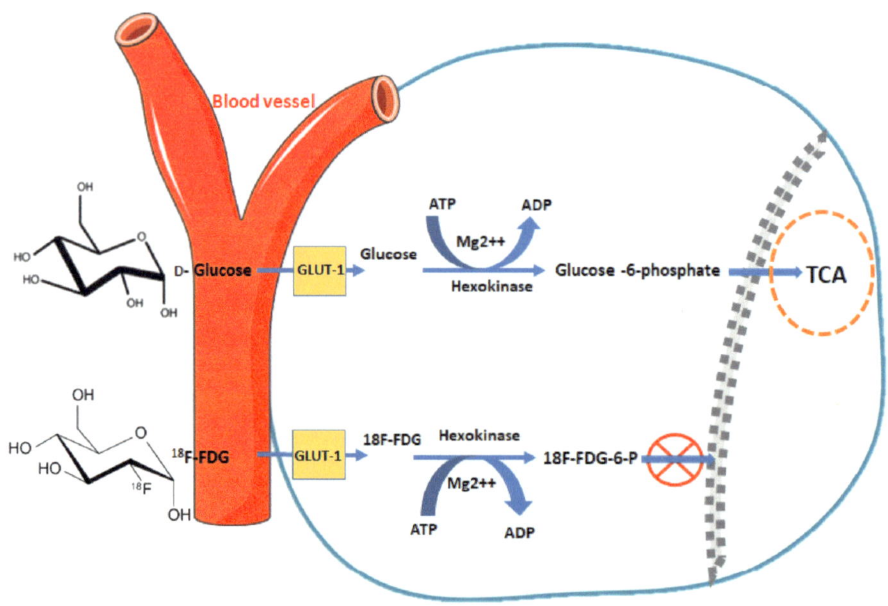

Figure 12.
Glucose and FDG transported inside cell, phosphorylated by hexokinase. ^{18}F-FDG-6-phosphate did not metabolized further but glucose-6-phosphate continue metabolism in cell mitochondria. Tumor cell, ischemic myocytes and macrophage acquired more ^{18}F-FDG [45].

leukocytes (mainly neutrophil) are frequently used complexes for infection and sterile inflammation site studies. Physiologically, autologous leukocytes chemotactically migrate towards pathogens in fact studies extended the use of leukocytes for radiolabeling that not only invade pathogens but also diagnose infection foci. At least 2000 or more leukocyte per microliter should be labeled for better quality image [40]. Labeled leukocytes were mostly neutrophil so that these complexes more sensitive to the neutrophil mediated infections. The uptake and rate of migration of radiolabelled cells depends upon the site of infection, virulence, stage of infection, kind of pathogen, upon antibiotic therapy and angiogenesis of tissues [41].

Ex-vivo labelling of ^{111}In- oxyquninoline with leukocytes was initiated by McAfee and Thakur [42]. The ^{111}In-oxine was neutral, lipid soluble, non-specific blood cells labeling agent that passively penetrate through bilayer membrane and bind with cytosol component (lactoferrin; iron bounded protein released by neutrophil). The lactoferrin bind with indium more firmly than oxine and free oxine (8-hydroxyquinoline) leave the cell environment. Scintigraphy using ^{111}In-oxine (8-hydroxyquinoline) with labeled leukocytes (WBCs) were the clinically proved agent of choice for detecting infection foci accurately [43, 44].

Approximately after 1 hour of injection, about 60% radioactivity of indium labeled leukocytes were found in the lungs and if not damaged migrate to liver, spleen, bone marrow and reticuloendothelial system. In case of infection, radiolabeled WBCs accumulate at the site of infection due to chemotactic attraction of biofilms and other soluble products of bacteria. The reason for the regular usage of ^{111}In- leukocyte for tumor imaging were its stability, normal body distribution and complementary bone marrow imaging as shown in **Figure 13**. The cons of complex are its lower sensitivity in infection that cannot elicit the neutrophil response e.g. tuberculosis and about 18 to 30 h delay in injection administration and imaging [40].

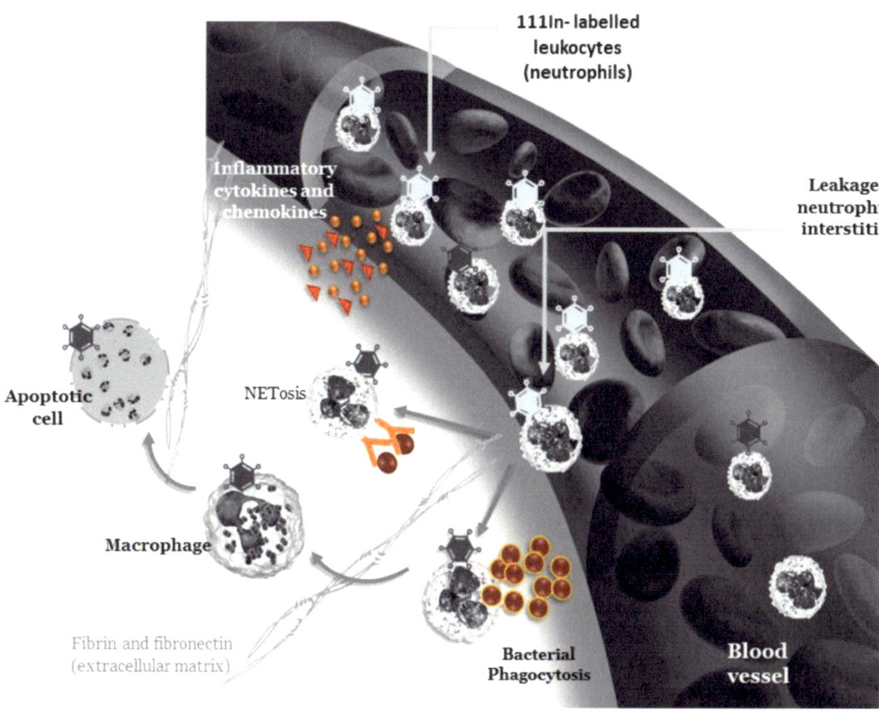

Figure 13.
Depiction of tumor cell microenvironment. ^{111}In-oxine labeled with leukocytes. Leukocytes move within blood stream and act as first line of defense. Attached radiotracer (^{111}In) image tumor cell microenvironment [45].

^{111}In-oxine labeled leukocytes preferably practiced for the diagnosis and therapy of inflammatory bowel disease, osteomyelitis, abdominal infection, diabetic foot, vascular prosthesis, pelvic sepsis, lung infection, fever of unknown origin, neurological infection, and endocarditis etc. Furthermore, for the ex-vivo radio-labeling sterile conditions should be taken because there was a possible risk of cross contamination that may be tainted with hepatitis B, C or HIV.

^{99m}Tc- exametazime (HMPAO) labeled with autologus leukocytes (predominantly neutrophils) follow the same pathway for infection and inflammation imaging as ^{111}In-oxine labeled leukocytes. Neutrophil, an important part of our innate immune system moved towards acute infection foci and invade pathogens [45]. Labelling of leukocytes followed by intervenously administration of radiolabelled complex, due to inflammatory cytokines and chemokines; WBCs were attracted towards infection site. The ^{99m}Tc-leukocyte detect abnormalities soon after the injection and image not only reticuloendotelial system but also visualize urinary tract, bowl and gall bladder. Limitation includes the short half life of ^{99m}Tc and delayed bone marrow imaging (2 to 3 days between leukocyte imaging and bone marrow imaging) [40].

Platelets; an important part of thrombus formation, when **labeled with ^{111}In** can follow simple cell migration mechanism to incorporate inside active thrombus formation so that easily picturize the thrombus formation. **Heat damaged ^{99m}Tc-RBCs** taken up for the examination of splenic nodule tissue formed after splectomy. During circulation of old and new RBCs, the old and damaged one was sequenter in the spleen. In same way heat damaged labeled RBCs sequenter inside spleen and imaged accessory spleen tissues [45].

3. Infection imaging agents based on metabolic activities

Tumor cells have higher metabolic rate as compare to the normal body cells, this upreglate the metabolism of cells and trap more molecule per gram than normal somatic cells. Through different metabolic ways like enhanced glucose metabolism for harvesting more energy. Following mechanism involved in proliferating cell metabolism and

- Sugar metabolism
- Iron metabolism
- Amino acid metabolism
- Lipid metabolism
- Thymidine kinase activity and folic acid synthesis
- Imaging cell micro-environment through Hypoxia and acidic pH

3.1 Sugar metabolism

Cancerous cells proliferate rapidly and get more energy to fulfill physiological activities. Glucolysis is the preliminary energy driving metabolism. What would happen if the same metabolism used for imaging cell?

3.1.1 Deoxyglucose

An analogous molecule of glucose but not sugar it has one oxygen atom less than glucose. Fluorine (F- 18), a cyclotron based radionuclide labeled with glucose analogous (deoxyglucose) through nucleophilic reaction with mannos triflate (precursor) [2]. **^{18}F-FDG (fluorodeoxyglucose**) practice for clinical oncology since 1980s [46]. The fluorodeoxyglucose participate and transport inside cell by following the same pathway as glucose through glucose transporter; GLUT-1. This glucose transpoter GLUT-1 release in stress condition and a member of glucose regulating protein [45]. As said earlier deoxyglucose is a glucose analogous, so this analogous molecule metabolized by the same pathway as glucose and was trapped in place of glucose molecule and get phosphorylated (glycolysis) as shown in **Figure 12**.

Glucose-6-phosphate further participate in glycolysis but FDG-6- phosphate cannot metabolized (not being the subsequent substrate) as glycolytic enzyme glucose-6-phosphate isomerase (hexokinase) has strict structural and geometric demands so fluorine substituted; 2-oxy-2-fluoro-D-glucose trapped and accumulate inside cell cytoplasm (metabolic trapping) [44]. Remember that glucose and FDG compete for the same transporter GLUT-1, so higher glucose level may lower the uptake of FDG. The enzyme hexokinase may convert back fluoro-6-phosphate to FDG but cancerous cell have very low amount of this enzyme so this trapped molecule (^{18}FDG-6-PO_4) aid in-vivo study of homeostatic system without disturbing their function. ^{18}F-FDG is presently the most widely used PET tracer for imaging non-invasive malignant tissues that highly metabolized glucose [45].

The ^{18}F-fluorodeoxyglucose participate in imaging of osteomyelitis, spinal infections, endocarditis, infected joint prosthesis, diagnose FUO and diabetic foot infection. Limitation regarding ^{18}F-FDG use that it cannot differentiate between infection and sterile inflammation.

3.1.2 Sorbitol

Another alcohol soluble sugar; **sorbitol**, act as a metabolic substrate for bacterial specific imaging. Gram negative bacterial strains (*Klebsiella pneumoniae*, *Escherichia coli*, Yersinia pestis, Enterobacter spp., etc.) show promising findings but limited detection in case of Gram-positive bacteria and mammalian cancer cells. Sorbitol was taken up by the bacterial surface membrane transporter, then phosphorylated and metabolized in the same manner as glucose. Initially ^{18}F-FDG reduce to ^{18}F-FDS (fluorodeoxysorbitol) as shown in **Figure 14** than transported to bacterial cell environment where analogous glucose metabolism begin next [47]. Interesting fact is that mammalian cells did not have transporter for this sugar [43]. Moreover, ^{18}F-FDS act as promising agent in PET imaging for monitoring efficacy of antibacterial burden and proved to be safe for intravenous human use that determine radiation dosimetry and cell biodistribution [48].

3.2 Iron metabolism

For the development of new radiopharmaceuticals similarities with ferric ion (Fe^{+3}) was very important as iron is a fundamental part of our body and many iron binding proteins likewise transferrin, lactoferrin and ferritin transport and store iron in-vivo. $^{67}Ga^{++}$ ion produced at physiological pH its infection uptake is multifactorial since it shares similar chemical characteristic and biodistribution properties with ferric ion (Fe^{+3}). When ^{67}Ga- citrate administrated in blood plasma due to the increase cell permeability and blood flow about 90% activity exchange ligand

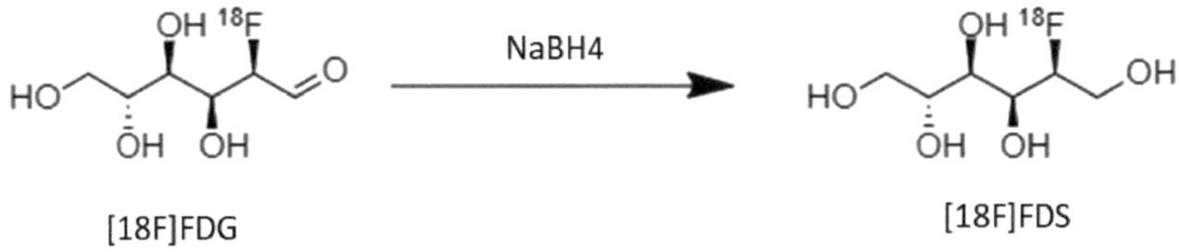

Figure 14.
Reduction reaction of 2-Deoxy-2-[^{18}F] fluoro-D-glucose to 2-Deoxy-2-[^{18}F] fluoro-D-sorbitol using $NaBH_4$ reducing agent.

with plasma protein in extracellular space. Therefore, iron atom always competes with radio-metal (^{67}Ga) for binding with plasma protein. ^{67}Ga-citrate exchange ligand with transferrin protein in cell plasma. Cancerous cells overexpress cell proliferation and metabolic activities, to meet the cell membrane receptors demand tumor and inflammatory cell membranes have ubiquitous membrane receptors on them. In fact, infinite transferrin receptors are getting to the cell having rapid cell growth and upregulated DNA synthesis (like tumor and inflammatory cells), thus ensuring more uptake of $^{67}Ga^{++}$.

^{67}Ga-citrate localize non-specifically at the site of infection where the ^{67}Ga-transferrin complex formed due to the leakage of plasma protein from blood vessel to extracellular space of inflamed tissues. The acidic environment of inflammatory interstitial tissue space has more lactoferrin another plasma protein secreted by stimulated or dead neutrophils, which subsequently tie with ^{67}Ga due to higher ionic attraction [2]. Another ^{67}Ga uptake mechanism seen in bacterial infection, a ^{67}Ga-avid, direct attachment of ^{67}Ga with bacterial siderophores (specific prokaryotic metal chelating peptides) [49]. Some gallium atoms also transported by circulating WBCs [40].

^{67}Ga-citrate used primarily for the diagnosis of spondylodiskitis, moreover for benign and neoplastic lymphomas particularly in evaluating staging, prognosis and follow up imaging of residual disease. Though ^{67}Ga-citrate not being specific for bacterial infection and replaced with ^{18}F-FDG/PET but still ^{67}Ga-citrate are widely used to identify the site of FUO and worthwhile in nuclear oncology (Hodgkin's and non- Hodgkin lymphoma) [2, 43, 50]. Disadvantages of ^{67}Ga may include its short physical half-life ($t_{1/2}$ = 68 min), uptake in inflammation and trauma [40].

3.3 Amino acid metabolism

Amino acids and proteins are the key elements in building block of life. Amino acid actively transport and uptake greaterly in the proliferating cancerous cells which reflects the increase synthesis of protein. Methionine, an essential natural occurring amino acid customize as l-[methyl-^{11}C] methionine and potentially used in PET oncology. Additionally tyrosine, another essential amino acid analog frequently used as radiolabelled tracer. As these tyrosine tracers not involved in protein synthesis [^{11}C] methyl-1-tyrosine,O-(2-[^{18}F] fluoroethyl)-L-tyrosine (FET), 1-[2-^{18}F] flourotyrosin, 1–4-[^{18}F] fluoro-m-tyrosin and 1-[3-^{18}F]-a-methyltyrosine (FMT), these analogs used in evaluating brain tumors, neuroendocrine tumors, prostate and pancreatic cancer uptake [45, 51, 52].

3.4 Lipid metabolism

The upregulation of glycolysis, iron and amino acid metabolism in cancerous cells also characteristically agitate the lipid production. During normal conditions production of triglycerides combined with long term energy reservoir. Cancerous cells do not manage the cell energy requirement with primary source; carbohydrates. So they preferentially employed lipid metabolism to meet energy requirement by producing more essential membrane phospholipids and phosphatidylcholine [46]. As a result two essential lipid production enzymes fatty acid synthase (FAS) and choline kinase (ChoK) overexpressed in lymphomas including breast, lung, colon, ovarian, and prostate cancers. So in lipid de novo synthesis FAS catalyze the acetic acid reaction for the synthesis of phospholipid phosphotidylcholine and choline kinase responsible for phosphocholine production as shown in **Figure 15**. Fatty acid radiolabelled analogs [^{11}C]- Acetate, [^{11}C]-Choline, [^{18}F]-Fluorodeshydroxycholine [^{18}F]-Choline, [^{18}F]-Flouoethycholine used in PET oncology imaging of brain tumors, liver tumors, prostate and breast malignancies [53, 54].

3.5 Thymidine kinase and folic acid synthesis pathway

Thymidine kinase; a metabolic substrate that catalyze the conversion reaction of nucleoside subunits to nucleotide units and then use these units in the synthesis of DNA. These labeled bacterial substrate initialize for SPECT [^{125}I]-FIAU and PET [^{124}I]-FIAU imaging. Thymidine based PET radiotracers [^{11}C] TdR, [^{18}F] FLT, [^{18}F] FMAU and [^{76}Br] FBAU [46, 57].

Folic acid; another metabolic salvage for nucleic acid synthesis (subsequently DNA synthesis) in prokaryotes. Para aminobenzoic acid (PABA) responsible for the folic acid production in microorganism and this substrate labeled with radiotracer [^{18}F]-PABA/PET. This radiofluronated analogues [^{18}F]-PABA holds potential for clinical translation in bacteria and poor attraction with mammalian cells [58].

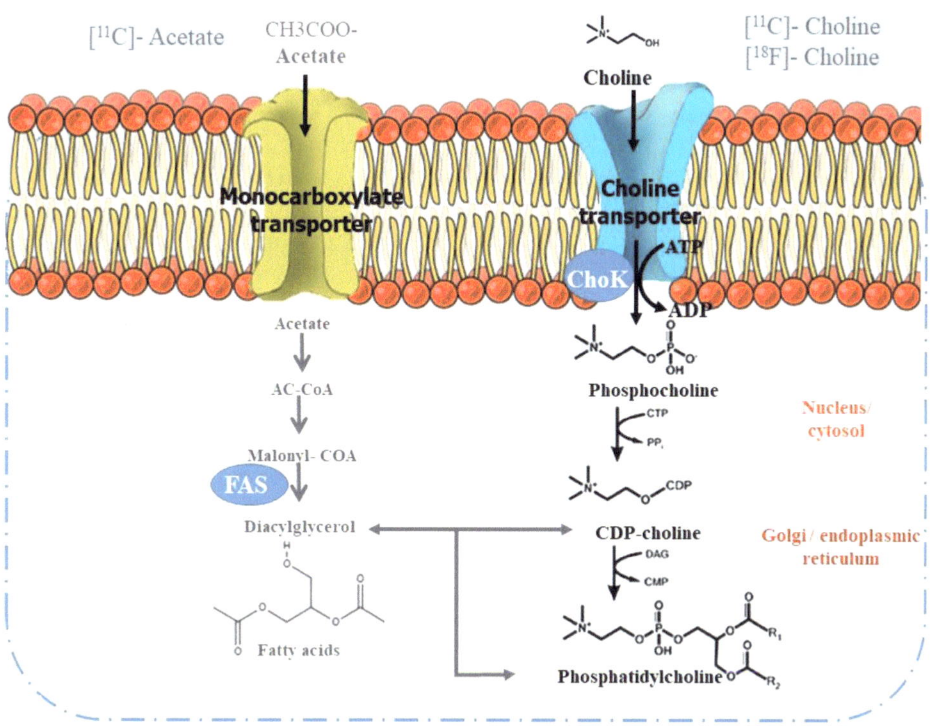

Figure 15.
De novo fatty acid synthesis mechanism using acetate substrate [55, 56].

3.6 Oxidative metabolism (tissue hypoxia)

Hyoxia, a phathophysiological condition portray deprived of adequate oxygen level in tissues. A normoxic cell have oxygen level 20–80 mmHg compared to hypoxic cell <3 mmHg. In malignancies, irregular vascularization cause ischemic hypoxia. The severity of cancerous hypoxia depend upon tumor phenotype for example cervical cancer has severe hypoxic injury. Hypoxia may alter the function in tumor microenvironment particularly angiogenesis, vasculogenisis, apoptosis and prospensity for metastasis [46].

Potential hypoxia selective PET radiotracer has been developed to evaluate tumor microenviroment.^{18}F-fluoromisonidazole (FMISO) and ^{64}Cu-[4-*N*-methyl-3-thiosemicarbazonato ligand] (ATSM) translated for hypoxia imaging [59].

4. Cell proliferation

Tumor specific radiolabeled drugs are now clinically approved for non-surgical treatment and molecular imaging of malignant growth of cells and definite modifications were implemented to make possible radionuclide therapy of cancerous cells. Uptake, delivery and retaining mechanisms of radiolabeled drugs in targeted tissues and organs involve many ways which are of particular importance [60]. Normally, cells and tissues maintain a consistency between cell proliferation and cell death. On the other side, carcinogenic cells promote cell growth. In addition, amplified mitotic rate, increased cell growth and reduced differentiation are responsible for enhanced cell propagation. Generally, progression rate of cancerous cells depends upon the differentiation levels of benign and malignant tissues that leads to advanced mitotic rates [61] (**Figure 16**).

The idea of localization of radiolabeled drugs at tumor sites is best described in terms of transformed physiology of specific proliferating cells. Such localization should take place in correlation with diseased parts of the body including external and internal regions of infected areas [63]. Tumor targeting involves a certain type of interaction between medication and its receptors at affected tissue site. Malignant tumors required excess quantity of nutrition and release certain receptors which, in contrast, used as carriers to distribute cytotoxic agents as shown in the above figure. Larger number of rapidly producing cells were compared with normal cells during cell cycle i.e. S-phase. Consequently, substrate requirement in the form of nucleotides for DNA synthesis was also increased. This nucleotide incorporation into DNA of tumor cells is determined using thymidine to measure the number of proliferated cells. ^{11}C-labeled thymidine has been utilized as PET radiotracer to image head and neck. Furthermore,

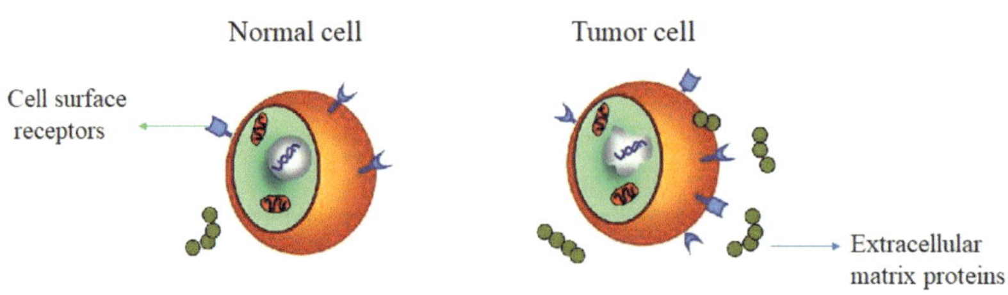

Figure 16.
Difference of cell surface receptors in normal and tumor cells [62].

targeted drug delivery systems necessitated drug localization and carriers within the desired organ.

In diseased patients, diagnosis and evaluation of therapeutic response is accomplished with positron emission tomography (PET). Studies based on this technology seek imaging mediators with eminent tumor selectivity and specificity for distinct attributes [64]. In 1950s, procedures were considered to estimate quantity of thymidine integrated into DNA of malignant tissues by using **^{3}H-Thymidine**. Meanwhile, in 1972, ^{11}C-labeled thymidine was evolved in molecular imaging to approximate cell growth. Nonetheless, rapid metabolic rate of this radiolabeled drug makes it less convenient for repetitive imaging practice.

^{18}F- 3′-deoxy-3′-fluorothymidine (FLT) is significantly developed radiotracer for molecular imaging techniques to investigate cell proliferation as it provides prolonged time interval so that there will be less quantity of labeled metabolites and scanning tissues will be cleared off catabolic waste. Transportation of FLT takes place into cell through distinct transporters and enzymatic action of thymidine kinase 1 (TK1) phosphorylated radioactive tracer into ^{18}F-FLT monophosphate that got trapped into cell. Moreover, PET images demonstrate additional phosphorylation into FLT-TP by enzyme thymidylate kinase. Reaction end products are then metabolically stuck within cells due to membrane impermeability and resistant to mortification.

FLT has greater potential to evaluate the status of malignant cells for therapeutic purposes. Diverse range of melanoma tissues i.e. breast, lung, head, neck, lymphoma and gastrointestinal have been analyzed by means of fluorine labeled thymidine [65]. Finally, ^{18}F-FLT is under evaluation and measurement of anticancer therapeutic response.

^{18}F-florouridine as a nucleoside analogue illustrates localization by cell proliferation but the radiopharmaceutical also incorporated into DNA and RNA of tumor tissues. **^{11}C-thymidine** was considered to observe multiplying tumor cells but prompted catabolic rates create hindrance in drug uptake volume and leads to complex imaging due to interfering catabolites (radiolabeled). **^{18}F-1-(2′-fluoro-2′-deoxy-β-D-ribofuranosyl) thymine (FMAU)**, a fluorine labeled analog of advanced stability with favorable results in animal cells. Phosphorylated complex incorporated into DNA to examine cell proliferation. Radioiodine I-131 & I-123 labeled **metaiodobenzylguanidine (MIBG)** represent the potent radioactive drug with diagnostic and therapeutic response to treat metastatic tumor. Even though, peptide receptors are now interchanging radiotherapy of neuroendocrine tumors, but the labeled drug still used to treat chromaffin tumors. Following ^{11}C-labeled amino acid analogs, **^{11}C-L-methionine and ^{11}C-5-hydroxytryptophane,** are used to visualize breakdown rates of cancer cells and imaging of different phases of thyroid tumors.

An analog of dihydroxyphenylalanine, **^{18}F-DOPA,** stored in brain tumor cells and exhibit amino acid transportation.^{18}F-labeled synthetic amino acids i.e. L-leucine derivatives, **^{18}F-fluoro-cyclobutyl carboxylic acid (FACBC)**, are preferentially firm and rigid with extended time frame of uptake by prostate tumor [66] (**Figure 17**).

^{18}F-fluoroethyl tyrosine (FET) localized in brain tumor cells and help to determine the type of therapeutic treatment and fate of proliferating tissues. ^{11}C and ^{18}F labeled pyrimidine analog, **2’-Fluoro-methyl-D-arabino-furanosyluracil (FMAU)** considered worthwhile for examining multiplying tumor cells. FMAU stored in the cancerous cells, phosphorylated and incorporated into DNA by enzymatic action of DNA polymerase with the potential to image DNA replication in normal and cancerous cells [68].

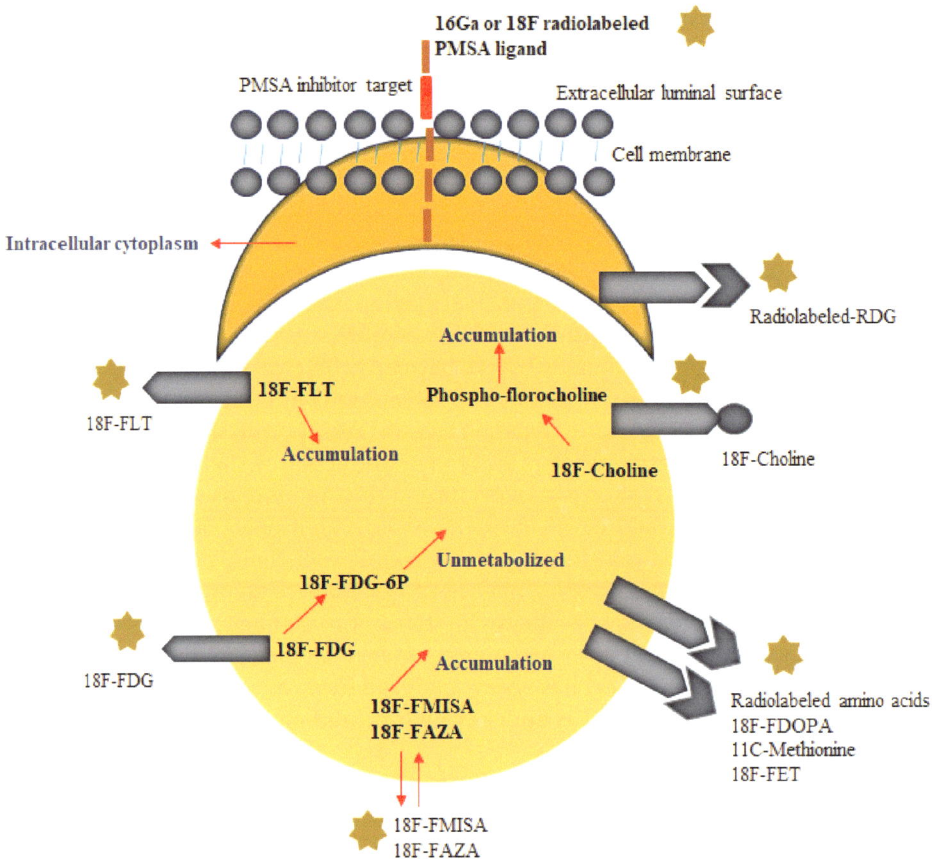

Figure 17.
Pathophysiological mechanisms of significant radiotracers used in investigation of malignant cells [67].

5. Specific receptor binding

Receptors are attachment sites for ligand molecules i.e. polypeptide hormones and neurotransmitters. In case of antigen–antibody complex formation, antigen expression on cell surface is considered a definite receptor site for antibody binding. Antigen fragments are present on the upper surface and within the cells or sometimes released into body fluids. Localization of definite receptor-binding radiotracers depends upon multiple factors such as blood clearance, affinity of the tracer & receptor and blood flow of the tumor tissue. Receptors are of various types with specificity of basic compound including peptides, steroid hormones, and antibodies.

5.1 Somatostatin receptors

Naturally, existing somatostatin (SST) complexes of peptide formation are of two types. One with 14 amino acids (SST_{14}) and other with 28 amino parts and designated as SST_{28}. In human beings, SST receptors have been recognized on cell surface of neuroendocrine region and on lymphocytes. Seglitide and somatuline are synthetically prepared somatostatin analogs with more stability than SST_{14} because the latter one join SSTR sub-types with equivalent association. To image growing SSTR cells, iodine labeled octreotide radioactive tracer pioneered the functioning of radiolabeled peptides [69] (**Figure 18**).

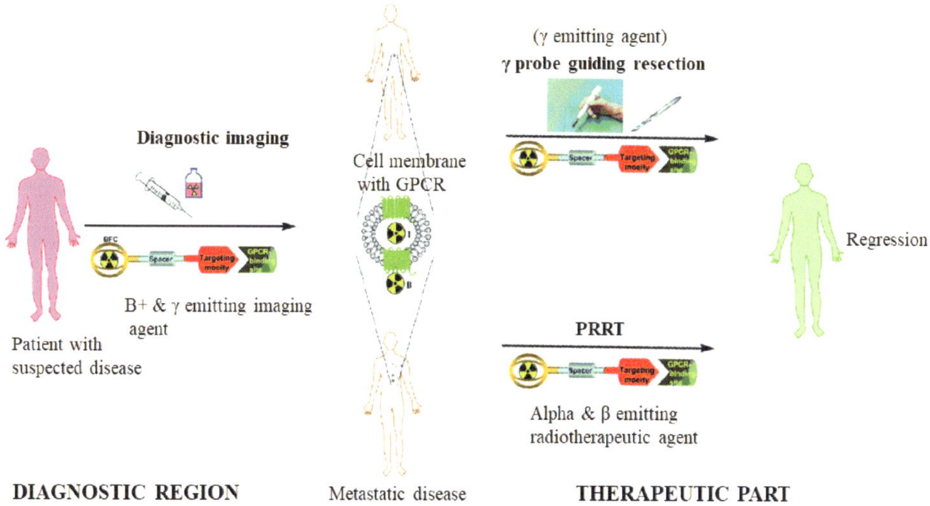

Figure 18.
Schematic representation of radiotheranostics using radiolabeled peptides [70].

- ^{111}**In-DTPA-pentetreotide**was developed with specific amounts of ^{111}In (10 μg) but showed short residing time as released from body circulation via kidneys (approximately 50% in 5 h). After that, ^{90}**Y-DOTA-octreotide** was formed with the similar capacity to bind proliferating cells revealing SSTR type 2.

- ^{99m}**Tc-P829 peptide** exhibited peculiar binding ability with SSTR types showing the potential to image rapidly growing cells. The radioactive product is FDA approved to image lung cancerous cells [71].

5.2 Vasoactive intestinal peptide (VIP) receptor

A 28 amino acid neuroendocrine moderator with diverse variety of biological activity in various cells and tissues. Although, receptors of cell membrane are extensively present along gastrointestinal tract. However, few receptor cells found on adenocarcinomas, malignant tumors, neuroblastomas, and pancreatic cancerous cells.

^{123}**I-VIP**was formulated with extraordinary activity ratio of radionuclide of about 200 MBq/μg of product to be specifically localized in liver, lung, pancreatic and gastrointestinal malignant cells [72].

5.3 Steroid hormone receptor

Steroid chemicals such as estrogen and progesterone have high binding affinity with intracellular receptors which are used to identify hormone dependent proliferating cells in case of breast cancer. Various types of hormonal analogs radiolabeled with PET imaging radiotracers. ^{18}**F-fluoro-estradiol (FES)**, with specificity for estrogen hormone, has revealed greater potential for analyzing metastatic tumor cells. ^{123}**I-methoxy-iodovinylestradiol** (radioactive ligand) was used to diagnose estrogen receptors in breast carcinogenic cells [73].

5.4 Low density lipoprotein (LDL) receptors

Plasma lipoprotein transports cholesterol towards adrenal gland that act as the substrate for synthesis of steroid hormone. ^{131}**I-iodomethyl-norcholeterol**

(NP 59) used to identify patients suffering from adrenal cortex. Cholesterol analogs, **^{131}I-iodocholestrol and ^{75}Se-iodomethyl-norcholestrol,** are under investigation for clinical advantages to detect malignant tissues. Besides N59, various iodine labeled hormonal products are undergo transportation and localization with the help of LDL receptors. A corticosteroid, Dexamethasone, reduce cholesterol uptake by controlling the production of ACTH [74].

6. Conclusion

Accumulation of radiopharmaceuticals at diseased cells through one or variety of localization mechanisms describes the specificity and efficacy of the tracer agent. The description of different localization mechanisms in above sections, helps in developing new radiopharmaceuticals for theranostics. However, the success of the radiopharmaceutical depends on the accumulation of radiopharmaceutical at specific target cells in term of per cent of injected dose per gram organ or tissue. According to the survey of literature, which has been cited in this chapter, different localization processes are quite promising but the receptor based localization of radiopharmaceuticals is the most successful nuclear medicine procedure both in diagnosis and therapeutic treatments of global fatal diseases.

Author details

Sana Komal[1], Sana Nadeem[1], Zahra Faheem[1], Arouma Raza[1], Komal Sarwer[1], Hijab Umer[1], Samina Roohi[2] and Syed Ali Raza Naqvi[1*]

1 Department of Chemistry, Government College University, Faisalabad-38000, Pakistan

2 Isotope Production Division, Pakistan Institute of Nuclear Science and Technology (PINSTECH), Nilore-Islamabad, Pakistan

*Address all correspondence to: draliraza@gcuf.edu.pk

IntechOpen

© 2020 The Author(s). Licensee IntechOpen. This chapter is distributed under the terms of the Creative Commons Attribution License (http://creativecommons.org/licenses/by/3.0), which permits unrestricted use, distribution, and reproduction in any medium, provided the original work is properly cited.

References

[1] Holland, J.P., *The Radiopharmaceutical chemistry of seldom-used radionuclides in nuclear medicine*, in *Radiopharmaceutical Chemistry*. 2019, Springer. p. 425-446.

[2] Vallabhajosula, S., R.P. Killeen, and J.R. Osborne, *Altered biodistribution of radiopharmaceuticals: role of radiochemical/pharmaceutical purity, physiological, and pharmacologic factors.* Semin Nucl Med, 2010. **40**(4): p. 220-41.

[3] Vallabhajosula, S. and A. Owunwanne, *Basis of Radiopharmaceutical Localization*, in *The Pathophysiologic Basis of Nuclear Medicine*. 2015, Springer. p. 45-68.

[4] Chamberlain, M.C. and J. Corey-Bloom, *Leptomeningeal metastases: 111Indium-DTPA CSF flow studies.* Neurology, 1991. **41**(11): p. 1765-1765.

[5] Bunker, S.R., et al., *Detection of Gastrointestinal Bleeding Sites: Use of In Vitro Technetium Tc 99m—Labeled RBCs.* JAMA, 1982. **247**(6): p. 789-792.

[6] Shaffer, E., P. McOrmond, and H. Duggan, *Quantitative cholescintigraphy: assessment of gallbladder filling and emptying and duodenogastric reflux.* Gastroenterology, 1980. **79**(5): p. 899-906.

[7] Hauser, W., et al., *Technetium-99m DTPA: a new radiopharmaceutical for brain and kidney scanning.* Radiology, 1970. **94**(3): p. 679-684.

[8] Brazil, R., *A barrier to progress: getting drugs to the brain.* Evaluation, 2020. **14**(47): p. 19.

[9] Welch, M., M. Adatepe, and E. Potchen, *An analysis of technetium (99mTcO4-) kinetics: The effect of perchlorate and iodide pretreatment.* The International journal of applied radiation and isotopes, 1969. **20**(6): p. 437-445.

[10] Ancri, D., et al., *Diagnosis of cerebral lesions by thallium 201.* Radiology, 1978. **128**(2): p. 417-422.

[11] Ancri, D. and J. Basset, *Diagnosis of cerebral metastases by thallium 201.* The British journal of radiology, 1980. **53**(629): p. 443-453.

[12] Jones, A.E., et al., *Brain scinTIGraphy with 99mTc pertechnetate, 99mTc polyphosphate, and 67Ga citrate.* Radiology, 1974. **112**(1): p. 123-130.

[13] Delmon-Moingeon, L.I., et al., *Uptake of the cation hexakis (2-methoxyisobutylisonitrile)-technetium-99m by human carcinoma cell lines in vitro.* Cancer research, 1990. **50**(7): p. 2198-2202.

[14] Arbab, A.S., et al., *Uptake of technetium-99m-tetrofosmin, technetium-99m-MIBI and thallium-201 in tumor cell lines.* Journal of Nuclear Medicine, 1996. **37**(9): p. 1551-1556.

[15] Rowe, S.P., et al., *Correlation of 99mTc-sestamibi uptake in renal masses with mitochondrial content and multi-drug resistance pump expression.* EJNMMI Research, 2017. **7**.

[16] Del Vecchio, S. and M. Salvatore, *99m Tc-MIBI in the evaluation of breast cancer biology.* European journal of nuclear medicine and molecular imaging, 2004. **31**(1): p. S88-S96.

[17] Moretti, J.-L., et al., *To use MIBI or not to use MIBI? That is the question when assessing tumour cells.* European journal of nuclear medicine and molecular imaging, 2005. **32**: p. 836-42.

[18] Hendrikse, N., et al., *Visualization of multidrug resistance in vivo.* European journal of nuclear medicine, 1999. **26**(3): p. 283-293.

[19] Ponto, J.A., *Mechanisms of radiopharmaceutical localization.* UNM College of Pharmacy, 2012. **16**(4).

[20] Vallabhajosula, S. and A. Owunwanne, *Pathophysiology and mechanisms of radiopharmaceutical localization*, in *The pathophysiologic basis of nuclear medicine*. 2006, Springer. p. 29-49.

[21] Tsopelas, C., *Radiotracers used for the scintigraphic detection of infection and inflammation.* The Scientific World Journal, 2015. **2015**.

[22] Miot-Noirault, E., et al., *Scintigraphic in vivo assessment of the development of pulmonary intravascular macrophages in liver disease: experimental study in rats with biliary cirrhosis.* Chest, 2001. **120**(3): p. 941-947.

[23] Schindl, M.J., et al., *The adaptive response of the reticuloendothelial system to major liver resection in humans.* Annals of surgery, 2006. **243**(4): p. 507.

[24] Saha, G.B., et al., *Experience with technetium-99m albumin colloid kit for reticuloendothelial system imaging.* Journal of nuclear medicine technology, 1986. **14**(3): p. 149-151.

[25] Hunt, A., et al., *Preparation of Tc-99m-macroaggregated albumin from recombinant human albumin for lung perfusion imaging.* European journal of pharmaceutics and biopharmaceutics, 2006. **62**(1): p. 26-31.

[26] Gandhi, S.J., et al., *Tc-99m macro aggregated albumin scintigraphy - indications other than pulmonary embolism: A pictorial essay.* Indian journal of nuclear medicine : IJNM : the official journal of the Society of Nuclear Medicine, India, 2013. **28**(3): p. 152-162.

[27] Levine, G., *Tc-99m MAA: A Model for Administering the Desired Number of Particles for Pulmonary Perfusion Studies.* Journal of Nuclear Medicine Technology, 1980. **8**(1): p. 33-36.

[28] Gandhi, S.J., et al., *Tc-99m macro aggregated albumin scintigraphy– Indications other than pulmonary embolism: A pictorial essay.* Indian Journal of Nuclear Medicine: IJNM: The Official Journal of the Society of Nuclear Medicine, India, 2013. **28**(3): p. 152.

[29] Som, P., et al., *Detection of gastrointestinal blood loss with 99mTc-labeled, heat-treated red blood cells.* Radiology, 1981. **138**(1): p. 207-209.

[30] Ehrlich, C.P., et al., *Splenic scintigraphy using Tc-99m-labeled heat-denatured red blood cells in pediatric patients: concise communication.* Journal of nuclear medicine: official publication, Society of Nuclear Medicine, 1982. **23**(3): p. 209-213.

[31] Khandan, A., E. Karamian, and M. Bonakdarchian, *Mechanochemical synthesis evaluation of nanocrystalline bone-derived bioceramic powder using for bone tissue engineering.* Dental Hypotheses, 2014. **5**(4): p. 155.

[32] Czernin, J., N. Satyamurthy, and C. Schiepers, *Molecular mechanisms of bone 18F-NaF deposition.* Journal of Nuclear Medicine, 2010. **51**(12): p. 1826-1829.

[33] Silberstein, E.B. *Systemic radiopharmaceutical therapy of painful osteoblastic metastases.* in *Seminars in radiation oncology*. 2000. Elsevier.

[34] Bokhari, S., et al., *99mTc-pyrophosphate scintigraphy for differentiating light-chain cardiac amyloidosis from the transthyretin-related familial and senile cardiac amyloidoses.* Circulation: Cardiovascular Imaging, 2013. **6**(2): p. 195-201.

[35] Russell, R.G.G., *Bisphosphonates: mode of action and pharmacology.* Pediatrics, 2007. **119**(Supplement 2): p. S150-S162.

[36] Dewanjee, M.K. and P.C. Kahn, *Mechanism of localization of*

99mTc-labeled pyrophosphate and tetracycline in infarcted myocardium. J Nucl Med, 1976. **17**(7): p. 639-46.

[37] Mulligan, J.S., P.W. Blue, and J.A. Hasbargen, *Methods for measuring GFR with technetium-99m-DTPA: an analysis of several common methods.* J Nucl Med, 1990. **31**(7): p. 1211-9.

[38] Taylor, A.T., *Radionuclides in nephrourology, part 1: radiopharmaceuticals, quality control, and quantitative indices.* Journal of Nuclear Medicine, 2014. **55**(4): p. 608-615.

[39] Elgazzar, A.H., *Basis of Radiopharmaceutical Localization*, in *Synopsis of Pathophysiology in Nuclear Medicine*. 2014, Springer. p. 27-40.

[40] Palestro, C.J., *Radionuclide Imaging of Musculoskeletal Infection: A Review.* J Nucl Med, 2016. **57**(9): p. 1406-12.

[41] Signore, A., et al., *Clinical indications, image acquisition and data interpretation for white blood cells and anti-granulocyte monoclonal antibody scintigraphy: an EANM procedural guideline.* Eur J Nucl Med Mol Imaging, 2018. **45**(10): p. 1816-1831.

[42] McAfee, J.G. and M.L. Thakur, *Survey of radioactive agents for in vitro labeling of phagocytic leukocytes. I. Soluble agents.* J Nucl Med, 1976. **17**(6): p. 480-7.

[43] Ordonez, A.A. and S.K. Jain, *Pathogen-Specific Bacterial Imaging in Nuclear Medicine.* Semin Nucl Med, 2018. **48**(2): p. 182-194.

[44] Salmanoglu, E., S. Kim, and M.L. Thakur, *Currently Available Radiopharmaceuticals for Imaging Infection and the Holy Grail.* Semin Nucl Med, 2018. **48**(2): p. 86-99.

[45] Elgazzar, A.H., *Synopsis of pathophysiology in nuclear medicine.* 2014.

[46] Strauss, H.W., *Nuclear oncology : pathophysiology and clinical applications.* 2013.

[47] Li, Z.-B., et al., *The Synthesis of 18F-FDS and Its Potential Application in Molecular Imaging.* Molecular Imaging and Biology, 2008. **10**(2): p. 92-98.

[48] Zhu, W., et al., *Biodistribution and Radiation Dosimetry of the Enterobacteriaceae-Specific Imaging Probe [18F]Fluorodeoxysorbitol Determined by PET/CT in Healthy Human Volunteers.* Molecular Imaging and Biology, 2016. **18**(5): p. 782-787.

[49] Welling, M.M., et al., *An update on radiotracer development for molecular imaging of bacterial infections.* Clinical and Translational Imaging, 2019. **7**(2): p. 105-124.

[50] Palestro, C.J., *The current role of gallium imaging in infection.* Seminars in Nuclear Medicine, 1994. **24**(2): p. 128-141.

[51] Wester, H.J., et al., *Synthesis and radiopharmacology of O-(2-[18F] fluoroethyl)-L-tyrosine for tumor imaging.* J Nucl Med, 1999. **40**(1): p. 205-12.

[52] Sharma, R., et al., *A comparison study of (11)C-methionine and (18) F-fluorodeoxyglucose positron emission tomography-computed tomography scans in evaluation of patients with recurrent brain tumors.* Indian journal of nuclear medicine : IJNM : the official journal of the Society of Nuclear Medicine, India, 2016. **31**(2): p. 93-102.

[53] Hodolic, M., *Role of (18)F-choline PET/CT in evaluation of patients with prostate carcinoma.* Radiology and oncology, 2011. **45**(1): p. 17-21.

[54] Welle, C.L., et al., *11C-Choline PET/CT in Recurrent Prostate Cancer and Nonprostatic Neoplastic Processes.* RadioGraphics, 2016. **36**(1): p. 279-292.

[55] Cornell, R. and N. Ridgway, *CTP: phosphocholine cytidylyltransferase: Function, Regulation, and Structure of an amphitropic enzyme required for membrane biogenesis.* Progress in lipid research, 2015. **59**.

[56] Spick, C., K. Herrmann, and J. Czernin, *Evaluation of prostate cancer with 11C-Acetate PET/CT.* Journal of Nuclear Medicine, 2016. **57**: p. 30S–37S.

[57] Smith, G., et al., *Synthesis and evaluation of nucleoside radiotracers for imaging proliferation.* Nucl Med Biol, 2012. **39**(5): p. 652-65.

[58] Zhang, Z., et al., *Positron Emission Tomography Imaging with 2-[(18) F]F- p-Aminobenzoic Acid Detects Staphylococcus aureus Infections and Monitors Drug Response.* ACS Infect Dis, 2018. **4**(11): p. 1635-1644.

[59] Xu, Z., et al., *(18) F-Fluoromisonidazole in tumor hypoxia imaging.* Oncotarget, 2017. **8**(55): p. 94969-94979.

[60] Bae, Y.H. and K. Park, *Targeted drug delivery to tumors: myths, reality and possibility.* Journal of controlled release, 2011. **153**(3): p. 198.

[61] Livingston, R.B., et al., *In vitro determination of thymidine-3H labeling index in human solid tumors.* Cancer research, 1974. **34**(6): p. 1376-1380.

[62] Abdalla, A.M.E., et al., *Engineered nanoparticles: thrombotic events in cancer.* Nanoscale, 2014. **6**(23): p. 14141-14152.

[63] Winchell, H.S. *Mechanisms for localization of radiopharmaceuticals in neoplasms*. Elsevier.

[64] Wells, P., et al., *Assessment of proliferation in vivo using 2-[11C] thymidine positron emission tomography in advanced intra-abdominal malignancies.* Cancer research, 2002. **62**(20): p. 5698-5702.

[65] Shields, A.F., *PET imaging of tumor growth: not as easy as it looks.* Clinical cancer research, 2012. **18**(5): p. 1189-1191.

[66] Chen, X. and S. Wong, *Cancer theranostics*. 2014: Academic Press.

[67] Moreau, A., et al., *Contribution of Different Positron Emission Tomography Tracers in Glioma Management: Focus on Glioblastoma.* Frontiers in Oncology, 2019. **9**.

[68] Sun, H., et al., *Imaging DNA synthesis with [18 F] FMAU and positron emission tomography in patients with cancer.* European journal of nuclear medicine and molecular imaging, 2005. **32**(1): p. 15-22.

[69] Patel, Y.C., et al., *The somatostatin receptor family.* Life sciences, 1995. **57**(13): p. 1249-1265.

[70] Fani, M., P.K. Peitl, and I. Velikyan, *Current status of radiopharmaceuticals for the theranostics of neuroendocrine neoplasms.* Pharmaceuticals, 2017. **10**(1): p. 30.

[71] Virgolini, I., et al., *Somatostatin receptor subtype specificity and in vivo binding of a novel tumor tracer, 99mTc-P829.* Cancer Research, 1998. **58**(9): p. 1850-1859.

[72] Virgolini, I., et al., *Cross-competition between vasoactive intestinal peptide and somatostatin for binding to tumor cell membrane receptors.* Cancer research, 1994. **54**(3): p. 690-700.

[73] Horti, A.G., et al., *18F-ASEM, a radiolabeled antagonist for imaging the α7-nicotinic acetylcholine receptor with PET.* Journal of Nuclear Medicine, 2014. **55**(4): p. 672-677.

[74] Pérez-Medina, C., et al., *PET imaging of tumor-associated macrophages with 89Zr-labeled high-density lipoprotein nanoparticles.* Journal of Nuclear Medicine, 2015. **56**(8): p. 1272-1277.

Chapter 6

Radiolabelled Nanoparticles for Brain Targeting

Dimple Sethi Chopra

Abstract

Tumors like glioblastoma are inaccessible due to blood brain barrier. The permeability of radioisotopes can be improved by conjugating them with nanoparticles. The most common malignant adult brain tumor is glioblastoma, which has very poor patient prognosis. The mean survival for highly proliferative glioblastoma is only 10–14 months despite an aggressive radiotherapy and chemotherapy following debulking surgery. β^- particle emitters like ^{131}I, ^{90}Y, $^{186/188}Re$, and ^{177}Lu have been coupled with nanoparticles and used for treatment of glioblastoma. These radiopharmaceutical compounds have resulted in a stabilization and improvement of the neurological status with minimal side effects. Similarly, α particle emitters like ^{213}Bi, ^{211}At, and ^{225}Ac are an innovative and interesting alternative. Alpha particles deliver a high proportion of their energy inside the targeted cells within a few micrometers from the emission point versus several millimeters for β^- particles. Thus, α particles are highly efficient in killing tumor cells with minimal irradiation of healthy tissues and permits targeting of isolated tumor cells. This has been confirmed by subsequent clinical trials which showed better therapeutic efficacy and minimal side effects, thus opening a new and promising era for glioblastoma medical care using α therapy.

Keywords: radioisotopes, nanoparticles, brain targeting, glioblastoma, blood brain barrier, theranostics

1. Introduction

Nuclear medicine involves use of radioactive atoms for diagnosis and/or therapy. For therapeutic purposes, to obtain specific irradiation of tumor cells, radioactivity is attached to a pharmaceutical molecule that binds to specific molecules expressed on the target tumor cells. This specific radioactive molecule is known as radiopharmaceutical. The pharmacological specific component of a therapeutic radiopharmaceutical can be based on the target protein structure which may include peptides or monoclonal antibodies, or molecular structures like nanoparticles [1]. The radioactive part may consist of massive particle emitters capable of delivering ionizing energy locally as Auger electrons, or β^- or α particles. Auger electrons are low-energy electrons that emit localized irradiation, few nanometers around the emission point with high biological effects. Beta-negative particles have a comparatively low linear energy transfer (LET) and emit their energy over a few millimeters in comparison to alpha particles. The choice of the radionuclide is based upon the size of the tumor. For example, yttrium-90 emits a long-range beta emission and could be useful for proliferating tumors of large size, while lutetium-177 having a short range emission could be used for treatment retreating tumors of small size. Alpha particles deliver a high fraction of their energy inside the targeted cells, leading to highly efficient killing. This makes them suitable for targeting cells of isolated tumor and minimal residual disease [2, 3].

Radioimmunotherapy, radiopeptide therapy and radionanoparticles are three important strategies of nuclear medicine for glioblastoma therapy. The four main prerequisites for successful radionuclide therapy for glioblastoma are selection of an appropriate target (integrin, tenascin, cadherin, EGFR, chemokine receptors or neurokinin receptors), physicochemical properties of the radionuclide, physicochemical properties of the targeting vector and its size [4]. For therapeutic purposes, nuclear medicine practitioners typically use β^- particle emitters like ^{131}I, ^{90}Y, $^{186/188}Re$, and ^{177}Lu. These radioisotopes have been coupled with nanoparticles, monoclonal antibodies, or peptides for treatment of glioblastoma. These radiopharmaceuticals have resulted in maintenance and/or improvement of the neurological status with only short-term side effects. The evidence for glioblastoma targeted radiotherapy has not only proven for β^- particle emitters but also for α particle emitters. ^{213}Bi, ^{211}At, and ^{225}Ac are some of the particle emitters which are recently attracting the interest of the scientific community. They are capable of delivering high amount of their energy within few micrometers close to their emission point in comparison to some few millimeters for β^- particles. The α particles have been found highly efficient in killing tumor cells with minimal irradiation of healthy tissues and permits targeting of isolated tumor cells [1, 5].

2. Understanding WHO Classification of CNS tumors

Gliomas are the most frequent, very diverse group of intrinsic tumors of the central nervous system and are conventionally classified in harmony to their microscopic alikeness with recognized cells of origin according to glial precursor cell families. Major groups consist of diffuse gliomas, categorized by widespread growth into the adjoining CNS parenchyma, and more confined "nondiffuse" gliomas, with pilocytic astrocytoma and ependymomas [6]. The fourth edition of the WHO Classification of CNS tumors published in 2016 has essentially changed the classification of diffuse gliomas. These tumors are presently defined based on presence/absence of IDH mutation and 1p/19q codeletion. It can be attributed to massive expansion of knowledge on molecular alterations in tumors of the central nervous system (CNS) [2]. Until now, tumors were defined based on their histology. Any molecular information was mainly provided as supplementary information within histologically defined categories. Current advances in the molecular conceptualization of gliomas recommend some probable reasons for the failure of targeted therapies in gliomas. Specially, the histologic-based glioma categorization comprises of multiple molecular subtypes with discrete biology, usual history, and diagnosis. These observations have resulted in improvement in diagnosis and classification by the World Health Organization [7]. These perceptions regarding glioma biomarkers and subtypes highlight several clinical challenges. Firstly, the field is witnessing the struggle of reconsidering the results of previous studies and retrospective data using the new classifications to explain prognostic assessments and treatment recommendations for patients. Secondly, the new classification requires changes in the design and stratification of future clinical trials. Hence, these observations offer the required framework for the growth and evaluation of novel targeted therapies for specific glioma subtypes [2, 8].

Drug delivery to tumor can be monitored using nuclear medicine imaging techniques like single-photon emission computed tomography (SPECT), positron-emission-tomography (PET). In single-photon emission computed tomography (SPECT), a gamma-emitting tracer allows for three dimensional visualization of the drug [9]. The radioisotope is either administered with the drug or directly bound to the biologically active molecule such as siRNA, so that their volume of distribution can be determined easily. Accurate anatomic estimates can be obtained by combining SPECT with CT or MRI. This approach is less expensive in comparison to other nuclear medicine imaging modalities [10]. Conventional SPECT suffer from poor limitation. However, recent advances involving pinhole-SPECT has improved the resolution to millimeter level [11].

Another promising modality for imaging drug delivery to tumor is positron-emission-tomography (PET). PET tracers are administered with the drug or are bound to the carrier like nanoparticles [12]. The PET scan can be correlated with CT scan in order to determine path of diffusion of tracer.

Similar to gadolinium and SPECT contrast agents, PET tracers can be infused concurrently with drug or bound to the delivery system, such as nanoparticles [12]. When PET is coupled with CT, molecular movement can be correlated with anatomy, with measurement of area of diffusion of tracer or tracer-incorporated carrier. PET imaging can estimate the borders of a tumor through the use of tracers that are derivatives of amino acid such as O-(2-[^{18}F]fluoroethyl)-L-tyrosine (FET) thus allowing precise assessment of drug distribution relative to tumor volume than MRI [13]. Limitations of PET and SPECT imaging include radiation exposure, the high cost, and short-lived nature of PET tracers. Another important limitation similar to gadolinium agents in MRI is the tracer has to directly couple to the delivery agent; otherwise the measurement of the area of diffusion is indirect. These limitations can be overcome by direct radiolabeling of nanoparticles [14].

3. Nanocarrier-mediated CNS delivery of diagnostic and therapeutic agents

Drug delivery across the BBB requires knowledge of both “barrier” and permeability properties of the brain endothelial cells. Transport across BBB may involve simple diffusion, facilitated diffusion, diffusion through aqueous pores, and active transport through protein carriers. In case of simple diffusion solute molecules travels along concentration gradient. Facilitated diffusion involves binding with specific membrane-traversing protein, coupled with movement along the concentration gradient. Charged ions and solutes cross the BBB by diffusion through aqueous pores. Active transport of solutes through protein carrier against concentration gradient involves expenditure of ATP. The presence of large number of mitochondria in the endothelial cells is thought to provide the required energy in form of ATP [15]. This mechanism involves an alteration in the affinity of a carrier for the solute molecules as it travels across the BBB. While designing nanocarrier mediated CNS delivery, transporter systems involved in ferrying essential molecules such as glucose are of utmost importance. These systems can be employed for delivery of potential nanotheranostics across the BBB. There are five types of sodium-independent glucose transporters (GLUT) which transport 2-deoxyglucose, 3-O-methylglucose, mannose, galactose and glucose across the BBB. The most important being 45–55 kDa glycosylated protein GLUT-1. It is mostly present in endothelial cells of arterioles, venules and capillaries, wherein it facilitates movement of D-glucose from the peripheral circulation into the brain. Other worth mentioning glucose transporters are GLUT-3 in brain neurons and GLUT-5 in microglial cells in the brain. They transport 2-deoxyglucose, 3-O-methylglucose, mannose, galactose and glucose across the BBB [16].

Another significant transport system that works in an analogous manner is P-glycoprotein multiple drug resistant protein (P-gp, MDR1). It has been comprehensively investigated as a possible carrier for drug delivery. This efflux transporter is usually expressed on luminal surface of endothelial cells, astrocytes and microglial cells. It prevents toxins from gaining entry into the brain parenchyma [17, 18]. Anticancer agents like Vinca alkaloids, anthracyclines, and taxanes are substrates for MDR1 are transported by Pgp. It limits their accumulation in the brain. Recently, it has been found that MDR1 regulation is altered by various disease conditions, and, in turn, diseases of the brain influence MDR1 expression [19, 20]. The presence of large number of receptors at the surface of BBB can be utilized by potential nanocarriers for enhanced brain by coupling with receptor-specific molecules or analogues. A large number of molecules such as insulin, insulin-like growth factors (IGF-1 and IGF-2), leptins, and transferrin can be transported into the brain following receptor-mediated endocytosis [13]. The nanoparticles should be designed to bypass efflux transport systems present at the luminal side (such as MDR1). Instead, nanoparticles could be substrates of transport mechanisms enhancing the passage of specific molecules like GLUT-1, IGF-1, and IGF-2 across the BBB [21].

4. Paradigm shift in glioma diagnosis and treatment strategies

The WHO 2016 Classification of gliomas represents a paradigm shift as; for the first time, the definition of many of these neoplasms is partly based on genetic characteristics based on molecular markers. This was a major step forward toward a more precise diagnosis of gliomas and will in the course of time certainly facilitate improved therapeutic management of the patients suffering from these tumors. Diffuse gliomas are the most common intrinsic CNS neoplasms, found in adults. On the basis of histopathological analysis, these gliomas were conventionally diagnosed as diffuse astrocytomas (with glioblastoma as it is most common and malignant representative), oligodendrogliomas, or as tumors with a mixed astrocytic and oligodendroglial phenotype (oligoastrocytomas) [6]. Within these subgroups, a malignancy grade (WHO grade II, III or IV) was assigned based on the presence/absence of marked mitotic activity, necrosis and florid microvascular proliferation. The major change can be attributed to use of isocitrate dehydrogenase (IDH mutation) as a marker in diffuse glioma classification. The categorization of diffuse gliomas on the basis of genotype involves high incidence of point mutations in isocitrate dehydrogenase 1 and 2 (*IDH1/IDH2*) in WHO grade II and III astrocytomas, oligodendrogliomas, oligoastrocytomas and secondary glioblastomas. Lower grade neoplasms usually develop into secondary glioblastomas [8]. Hence, it became clear that tumors with identical histology can lead to different clinical outcome such as IDH-wildtype and IDH-mutant diffuse gliomas. Many histologically similar WHO grade II and WHO grade III IDH-wild type diffuse gliomas exhibit molecular characteristics like glioblastoma. These facts ultimately led to inclusion of IDH mutation as a crucial marker for glioma classification and the introduction of, genetically defined entities: diffuse astrocytoma, IDH-mutant; anaplastic astrocytoma, IDH-mutant; oligodendroglioma, IDH-mutant; anaplastic oligodendroglioma, IDH-mutant; and glioblastoma, IDH-mutant [7]. The molecular features of IDH-mutant glioma outweigh the histological diagnosis. A tumor having histology of an astrocytoma, detection of complete 1p/19q codeletion leads to diagnosis of oligodendroglioma. Likewise, for diffuse, IDH-mutant gliomas with oligodendroglial phenotype with complete absence of 1p/19q codeletion, the collective diagnosis may be astrocytoma, IDH-mutant and 1p/19q-non-codeleted [8]. Based on IDH mutation status, glioblastomas were reclassified as glioblastoma, IDH-wildtype and glioblastoma,

IDH-mutant. This latter category largely overlaps with what previously described secondary glioblastoma based on clinical, radiological and/or pathological evidence of a lower grade precursor lesion. Patients with a secondary glioblastoma or IDH-mutant glioblastoma are normally younger and have improved diagnosis than those with glioblastoma, IDH-wildtype. Analogous to grade II and grade III oligoastrocytic tumors, most glioblastomas with oligodendroglioma as explained in the WHO 2016 Classification are part of one of the genetic subgroups of diffuse glioma [7, 8]. One of the treatment strategies which are catching the attention of oncologist is nanotechnology. Nanoparticles (NP) are entities possessing diameter of 10–200 nm that hold great possibilities for design and biological applications. There has been an upsurge in development of nanodevices for diagnosis and treatment of brain tumors. Nanoparticles are carriers that can be designed to ferry one or more types of molecules to brain including MRI contrast agents, fluorescent and visible dyes, chemotherapeutic agents and photosensitizers. The targeted delivery of nanoparticles to brain tumors can be augmented by altering their particle size and surface characteristics [22, 23].

5. Multimodal tumor imaging and therapy

There has been moderate impact of targeted therapies in glioma. The therapies that have demonstrated a significant survival benefit for gliomas in Phase III clinical trials, including radiation, chemotherapy (temozolomide and PCV [procarbazine, lomustine, vincristine]), and tumor-treating fields, are based on nonspecific targeting of proliferating cells. An emerging field in glioblastoma nuclear medicine is use of radionanoparticles. These radioactive nanocarriers can be used passively as a simple tumor brachytherapy or can be actively used with a specific targeting to vectorize a large amount of radioactivity. The targeting is usually directed against a glioblastoma-specific antigen or receptor. Antigen targets, like epidermal growth factor receptor (EGFR), tenascin, or DNA histone H1 complex. Radiolabeled antibodies and peptides hold promise for molecular radiotherapy but are often limited by a low payload resulting in inadequate delivery of radioactivity to tumor tissue and, therefore, inadequate therapeutic effect and adverse effects due irradiation of normal tissues [24]. Song et al. developed a synthetic method of radiolabeling indium-111 (^{111}In) to epidermal growth factor (EGF)-gold nanoparticles (^{111}In-EGF-Au NP) with a high payload [25]. By using radiolabeled nanoparticles, comparatively higher payloads are obtained due to large surface area to volume ratio. This results in multivalent effect of nanoparticles, thus accommodating a large number of targeting ligands, such as antibodies, peptides or aptamers on a single nanoparticle. This facilitates maximal binding to the molecular target in vivo, thus enhancing delivery of radioactivity to target tissue with improved imaging and therapeutic efficacy. PEGylation of nanoparticles and alteration of their surface properties improves their stability and mean residence time in vivo [26]. It also permits loading a combination of imaging, radiotherapeutic and/or chemotherapeutic moieties for multimodal tumor imaging and therapy [27]. Antibodies, radiolabeled antibodies, antibody fragments or peptides because of their small size easily penetrate surrounding normal tissues. Loading onto nanoparticles limits their penetration through normal vasculature and capillaries, thus minimizing their side-effects [28].

Different nanocarriers such as metallofullerenes, liposomes, or lipid nanocapsules have been used to deliver radionanoparticle passively. A typical metallofullerene (^{177}Lu-DOTA-f-$Gd_3N@C_{80}$) radionanoparticles when administered by convection-enhanced delivery (CED) in brain tumor model showed an improved survival time of more than 2.5 times that of the control group [29]. Similarly liposomes loaded with beta-negative emitters such rhenium-186 and demonstrated promising results when administered by CED in an orthotopic glioblastoma rat model [30]. Lipid nanocapsules loaded with rhenium-188 in a rat orthotopic model showed a significant survival benefit after intratumoral stereotactic injection at day 6 and CED injection at day 12 [31].

A recent approach using radionanoparticles consists of an active targeting approach where the nanoparticles are functionalized and directed against a tumor target. The aim of this active targeting is to optimize the spatial localization of the radioactivity close to the tumor cells. As an example, lipid nanocapsules can be loaded with rhenium-188 and coupled to a monoclonal antibody directed against the CXCR4 antigen. These CXCR4-recognizing immune-nanoparticles irradiate the tumor cells and have been shown to increase efficacy in an orthotopic mouse model. Recurrence for the passive protocol was observed at 65 versus 100 days for the active targeting approach, and this appears to be the most effective therapy with the longest measured time to progression [32].

6. Neural stem cells functionalized with radiolabeled nanoparticles

Neural stem cells (NSCs) are increasingly being used as carriers for targeted delivery of therapeutics to glioblastoma. This requires multimodal dynamic in vivo imaging of NSC in the brain. Such type of technology is in development phase. Cheng et al. reported an innovative strategy for neural stem cell tracking in brain using silica nanoparticles via SPECT [33]. ^{111}In radioisotopes were conjugated to porous silica nanoparticles having large surface area. A series of nanomaterial characterization assays were performed to evaluate the modified mesoporous silica nanoparticles. Loading efficiency and viability of NSCs with ^{111}In-MSN complex was validated. Radiolabeled NSCs were administered to glioma-bearing mice via intracranial or systemic injection. SPECT and bioluminescence imaging were performed periodically after NSC injection. Histology and immunocytochemistry were performed to endorse the findings. ^{111}In-MSN complexes showed minimal toxicity to NSCs and adequate in vitro and in vivo stability. Phantom studies establish possibility of mesoporous silica nanoparticles for NSC imaging. It was found that decayed ^{111}In-MSN complexes exhibited significant fluorescent profiles in preloaded NSCs, thus validating ex vivo data. In vivo, SPECT images reveal actively migrating NSCs toward glioma xenografts in real time after both intracranial and systemic injection. This is in consonance with findings of histology, confocal microscopy and bioluminescence live imaging [33].

7. Conclusion

An urgent requirement for rapid detection and diagnosis of diseases has led to development of contrast agents and imaging techniques. The present challenge is for fast and complete imaging of tissues and lesion categorization that could be obtained by development of nontoxic contrast agents with longer blood circulation time. Nanotechnology provides apt solution to this problem. Nanoparticle based contrast agents have been employed in most biomedical imaging techniques like MRI, fluorescence imaging, CT, ultrasound, PET and SPECT. However, these imaging techniques have certain limitations. These can be overcome by use of multifunctional nanoplatforms to enhance safety, efficacy and theranostic attributes. The WHO 2016 Classification is a major step forward toward a more precise diagnosis of gliomas and will in the course of time certainly facilitate improved therapeutic management of the patients suffering from these tumors. The paradigm shift is IDH mutation as a marker in diffuse glioma classification and reclassification of glioblastoma. Novel drug delivery approaches have substantially influenced the glioblastoma treatment. There is urgent requirement of smart delivery systems for future therapies targeted to specific cells, dependent on intracellular delivery of agents impermeable to BBB. Polymer implants, convection enhanced delivery and degradable nanoparticles are some of the platform technologies for design of novel methods for treatment of glioblastoma. One strategy to optimize the efficacy of molecularly targeted radionuclide agents is to develop nanoparticle-based targeted delivery systems. An abundance of receptors at the surface of the BBB can be utilized by nanoparticles for enhanced brain uptake by coupling with receptor-specific molecules or analogues. The nanoparticles should be designed to bypass efflux transport systems present at the luminal side (such as MDR1). Instead, nanoparticles could be substrates of transport mechanisms enhancing the passage of specific molecules like GLUT-1, IGF-1, and IGF-2 across the BBB. Radiolabelled nanoparticles seem to be novel promising arsenal for potential neurotheranostics.

Author details

Dimple Sethi Chopra
Department of Pharmaceutical Sciences and Drug Research, Punjabi University, Patiala, India

*Address all correspondence to: dimplechopra24@yahoo.co.in

IntechOpen

© 2020 The Author(s). Licensee IntechOpen. This chapter is distributed under the terms of the Creative Commons Attribution License (http://creativecommons.org/licenses/by/3.0), which permits unrestricted use, distribution, and reproduction in any medium, provided the original work is properly cited.

References

[1] Bailly C, Vidal A, Bonnemaire C, Kraeber-Bodéré F, Chérel M, Pallardy A, et al. Potential for nuclear medicine therapy for glioblastoma treatment. Frontiers in Pharmacology. 2019;**10**:772. DOI: 10.3389/fphar.2019.00772

[2] Wesseling P, Capper D. WHO 2016 Classification of gliomas. Neuropathology and Applied Neurobiology. 2018;**44**:139-150

[3] Behling K, Maguire WF, Di Gialleonardo V, Heeb LEM, Hassan IF, Veach DR, et al. Remodeling the vascular microenvironment of glioblastoma with α-particles. Journal of Nuclear Medicine. 2016;**57**(11):1771-1777

[4] Cordier D, Krolicki L, Morgenstern A, Merlo A. Targeted radiolabeled compounds in glioma therapy. Seminars in Nuclear Medicine. 2016;**46**(3):243-249

[5] Behling K, Maguire WF, López Puebla JC, Sprinkle SR, Ruggiero A, O'Donoghue J, et al. Vascular targeted radioimmunotherapy for the treatment of glioblastoma. Journal of Nuclear Medicine. 2016;**57**(10):1576-1582. DOI: 10.2967/jnumed.115.171371

[6] Louis DN, Ohgaki H, Wiestler OD, et al. The 2007 WHO Classification of tumours of the central nervous system. Acta Neuropathologica. 2007;**114**:547-547

[7] Louis DN, Perry A, Reifenberger G, et al. The 2016 World Health Organization classification of tumors of the central nervous system: A summary. Acta Neuropathologica. 2016;**131**:803-820

[8] Chen R, Smith-Cohn M, Cohen AL, Colman H. Glioma subclassifications and their clinical significance. Neurotherapeutics. 2017;**14**(2):284-297. DOI: 10.1007/s13311-017-0519-x

[9] Merkel OM, Librizzi D, Pfestroff A, et al. In vivo SPECT and real-time gamma camera imaging of biodistribution and pharmacokinetics of siRNA delivery using an optimized radiolabeling and purification procedure. Bioconjugate Chemistry. 2009;**20**:174-182

[10] Sampson JH, Brady M, Raghavan R, et al. Colocalization of gadolinium-diethylene triamine pentaacetic acid with high-molecular-weight molecules after intracerebral convection-enhanced delivery in humans. Neurosurgery. 2011;**69**:668-676

[11] van der Have F, Vastenhouw B, Ramakers RM, et al. U-SPECT-II: An ultra-high-resolution device for molecular small-animal imaging. Journal of Nuclear Medicine. 2009;**50**:599-605

[12] Schluep T, Hwang J, Hildebrandt IJ, et al. Pharmacokinetics and tumor dynamics of the nanoparticle IT-101 from PET imaging and tumor histological measurements. Proceedings of the National Academy of Sciences of the United States of America. 2009;**106**:11394-11399

[13] Sirianni R, Carson R, Zheng M, et al. Development of dPET, a non-invasive imaging technique to measure the distribution of drugs after direct delivery to the brain. Journal of Nuclear Medicine. 2010;**51**:829-829

[14] Zhou J, Atsina KB, Himes BT, Strohbehn GW, Saltzman WM. Novel delivery strategies for glioblastoma. Cancer Journal. 2012;**18**(1):89-99. DOI: 10.1097/PPO.0b013e318244d8ae

[15] Lesniak MS, Brem H. Targeted therapy for brain tumours. Nature Reviews. Drug Discovery. 2004;**3**:499-508

[16] Yang H. Nanoparticle-mediated brain-specific drug delivery, imaging, and diagnosis. Pharmaceutical Research. 2010;**27**:1759-1771

[17] Neuwelt EA, Bauer B, Fahlke C, Fricker G, Iadecola C, Janigro D, et al. Engaging neuroscience to advance translational research in brain barrier biology. Nature Reviews. Neuroscience. 2011;**12**:169-182

[18] Maher F, Vannucci SJ, Simpson IA. Glucose transporter proteins in brain. The FASEB Journal. 1994;**8**:1003-1011

[19] Wong XY, Sena-Torralba A, Álvarez-Diduk R, Muthoosamy K, Merkoçi A. Nanomaterials for nanotheranostics: Tuning their properties according to disease needs. ACS Nano. 2020;**14**(3):2585-2627. DOI: 10.1021/acsnano.9b08133

[20] Nienhaus K, Wang H, Nienhaus GU. Nanoparticles for biomedical applications: Exploring and exploiting molecular interactions at the nano-bio interface. Materials Today Advances. 2020;**5**:100036. DOI: 10.1016/j.mtadv.2019.100036

[21] Biddlestone-Thorpe L, Marchi N, Guo K, Ghosh C, Janigro D, Valerie K, et al. Nanomaterial-mediated CNS delivery of diagnostic and therapeutic agents. Advanced Drug Delivery Reviews. 2012;**64**(7):605-613. DOI: 10.1016/j.addr.2011.11.014

[22] Orringer DA, Koo YE, Chen T, Kopelman R, Sagher O, Philbert MA. Small solutions for big problems: The application of nanoparticles to brain tumor diagnosis and therapy. Clinical Pharmacology and Therapeutics. 2009;**85**(5):531-534. DOI: 10.1038/clpt.2008.296

[23] Mohs AM, Provenzale JM. Applications of nanotechnology to imaging and therapy of brain tumors. Neuroimaging Clinics of North America. 2010;**20**(3):283-292. DOI: 10.1016/j.nic.2010.04.002. Review

[24] Steiner M, Neri D. Antibody-radionuclide conjugates for cancer therapy: Historical considerations and new trends. Clinical Cancer Research. 2011;**17**:6406-6416

[25] Song L, Falzone N, Vallis KA. EGF-coated gold nanoparticles provide an efficient nano-scale delivery system for the molecular radiotherapy of EGFR-positive cancer. International Journal of Radiation Biology. 2016;**92**(11):716-723. DOI: 10.3109/09553002.2016.1145360

[26] Gref R, Domb A, Quellec P, Blunk T, Muller RH, Verbavatz JM, et al. The controlled intravenous delivery of drugs using PEG-coated sterically stabilized nanospheres. Advanced Drug Delivery Reviews. 2012;**64**:316-326

[27] Eblan MJ, Wang AZ. Improving chemoradiotherapy with nanoparticle therapeutics. Translational Cancer Research. 2013;**2**:320-329

[28] Xing Y, Zhao JH, Conti PS, Chen K. Radiolabeled nanoparticles for multimodality tumor imaging. Theranostics. 2014;**4**:290-306

[29] Shultz MD, Wilson JD, Fuller CE, Zhang J, Dorn HC, Fatouros PP. Metallofullerene-based nanoplatform for brain tumor brachytherapy and longitudinal imaging in a murine orthotopic xenograft model. Radiology. 2011;**261**(1):136-143. DOI: 10.1148/radiol.11102569

[30] Phillips WT, Goins B, Bao A, Vargas D, Guttierez JE, Trevino A, et al. Rhenium-186 liposomes as convection-enhanced nanoparticle brachytherapy for treatment of glioblastoma. Neuro-Oncology. 2012;**14**(4):416-425. DOI: 10.1093/neuonc/nos060

[31] Vanpouille-Box C, Lacoeuille F, Belloche C, Lepareur N, Lemaire L,

LeJeune J-J, et al. Tumor eradication in rat glioma and bypass of immunosuppressive barriers using internal radiation with ^{188}Re-lipid nanocapsules. Biomaterials. 2011;**32**(28):6781-6790

[32] Séhédic D, Chourpa I, Tétaud C, Griveau A, Loussouarn C, Avril S, et al. Locoregional confinement and major clinical benefit of ^{188}Re-loaded CXCR4-targeted nanocarriers in an orthotopic human to mouse model of glioblastoma. Theranostics. 2017;7(18):4517-4536. DOI: 10.7150/thno.19403

[33] Cheng SH, Yu D, Tsai HM, Morshed RA, Kanojia D, Lo LW, et al. Dynamic in vivo SPECT imaging of neural stem cells functionalized with radiolabeled nanoparticles for tracking of glioblastoma. Journal of Nuclear Medicine. 2016;**57**(2):279-284